First Aid to Mental Illness

A Practical Guide for Patients and Caregivers

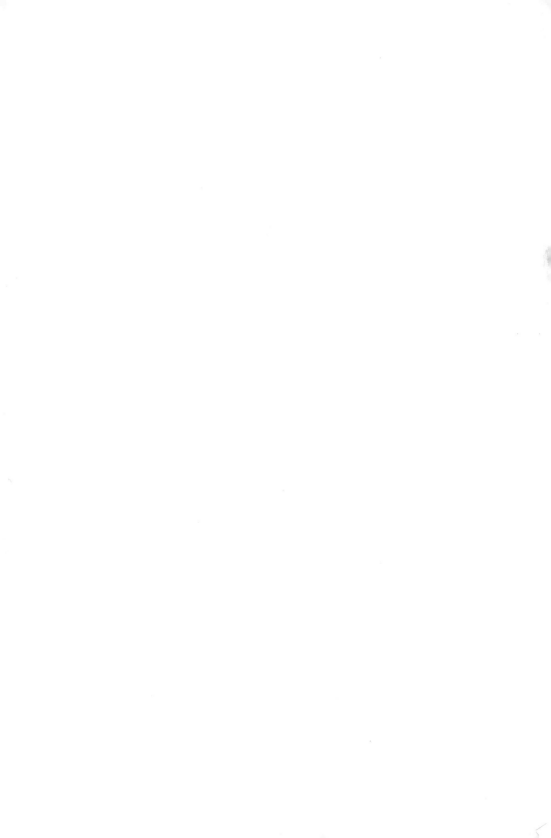

First Aid to Mental Illness

A Practical Guide for Patients and Caregivers

By

Michael G. Rayel, MD

SOAR DIME
Clarenville, NF

COPYRIGHT © 2002 by Michael G. Rayel, MD

All rights reserved. No part of this book shall be reproduced, stored in retrieval system, or transmitted by any means, electronic, mechanical, photocopying, recording, or otherwise, without written permission from the publisher. No patent liability is assumed with respect to the use of the information contained herein. Although every precaution has been taken in the preparation of this book, the publisher and author assume no responsibility for errors, inaccuracies, inconsistency, or omissions. All case scenarios are purely fictitious. Any resemblance to real people, either living or deceased, is entirely coincidental. Any slights against people or organizations are unintentional. Neither is any liability assumed for damages resulting from the use of information contained herein.

Note: This publication contains the opinions and ideas of its author. It is intended to provide helpful and informative material on the subject matter covered. It is sold with the understanding that the author and publisher are not engaged in rendering professional services in the book. If the reader requires personal assistance or advice, a competent professional should be consulted.

The author and publisher specifically disclaim any responsibility for any liability, loss or risk, personal or otherwise, which is incurred as a consequence, directly or indirectly, of the use and application of any of the contents of this book.

Published by:
    Soar Dime Limited
    PO Box 1834, Clarenville, NF
    Canada A0E1J0
    Phone: 709-466-5114 or 866-418-7277
    Fax: 709-466-2214
    E-mail: info@soardime.com Web: www.soardime.com

Printed in Canada by:
    Robinson-blackmore Printing and Publishing Limited

Canadian Cataloguing in Publication Data

Rayel, Michael G., 1963-
    First aid to mental illness: a practical guide for patients and caregivers / Michael G. Rayel

Includes bibliographical references and index.
ISBN 0-9687816-5-9

    1. Mental Illness--Treatment--Popular works. 2. First aid in illness and injury. I. title

RA 790.R392002   616.89'0252   C2002-901676-2

Acknowledgment

I sincerely thank my friends and colleagues Mona Romaine-Elliot, Evelyn Tilley, Wanda Green and John Mahar for their advice and constructive feedback. Because of your recommendations, the book has become more readable, practical and user-friendly. It has been mentally-stimulating and fun working with all of you. Once again, I thank Fred Manuel and Graham Manuel of The Writing Genius for excellent editing. Your attention to detail is superb.

I also acknowledge my wonderful grandparents, parents, brothers and sister. Without your constant love and selfless efforts, I would not be where I am today.

Most of all, I would like the world to know that my family – Gayzelle, my wife and our four wonderful children, Danielle, Joshua, Hannah, and Isaiah – is the engine that propels my profound desire to make a difference in other people's lives. Your love, laughter, and warm hugs constantly remind me that I need to reach out and share my blessings through our books.

Dedication

I sincerely dedicate this book to all patients and caregivers.

Table of Contents

About The Author	ix
Preface	xi
How To Use This Book	xiii
Chapter 1	
Why First Aid to Mental Illness?	1
Chapter 2	
The CARE Approach to First Aid	6
Chapter 3	
The HELP Method – Early Intervention for Caregivers	13
Chapter 4	
The HEAL Technique – Early Intervention for Patients	18
Chapter 5	
ABCs of First Aid	22
Chapter 6	
Basic Coping Skills to Help Deal with Mental Illness 1	28
Chapter 7	
Basic Coping Skills to Help Deal with Mental Illness 2	37
Chapter 8	
Depression	48
Chapter 9	
Mania or Mood Swings	59
Chapter 10	
Panic Attacks	68
Chapter 11	
Phobia	76
Chapter 12	
Obsessions and Compulsions	84
Chapter 13	
Emotional Difficulties After a Trauma	92
Chapter 14	
Anxiety	102
Chapter 15	
Psychosis	110
Chapter 16	
Excessive Drug or Alcohol Use	121
Chapter 17	
Eating Disorder	133
Chapter 18	
Dementia or Memory Loss	141

Chapter 19
    Grief and Bereavement   152
Chapter 20
    Commonly Asked Questions and Related Issues   160
Appendix
    Resources for Patients and Caregivers   167
References and Recommended Readings   177
Index   179

About The Author

Dr. Michael G. Rayel is an accomplished clinician, an administrator, and the author of several psychiatry books. Dr. Rayel, a Diplomate of the American Board of Psychiatry and Neurology and Certified in Clinical Psychopharmacology, trained in general psychiatry and psychodynamic psychotherapy at New York Medical College, geriatric psychiatry at New York University Medical Center, and forensic and correctional psychiatry at Harvard Medical School. He lives in Newfoundland, Canada.

Preface

Perceived by most people as a complex problem, mental illness requires a simplified and practical approach to dealing with its myriad problems. Many of my patients have lamented that, had they known what was going on with them emotionally, they could have done "something" about it during the early phase of the illness. Based on discussion with my patients and their caregivers, two issues have always caught my attention. First, they were unable to recognize the ongoing emotional difficulty. And secondly, they did not know the basic approach once they became aware of the change.

Since there is a dearth of first aid approaches to mental illness, I decided to devise user-friendly and easy-to-remember strategies to help patients and caregivers recognize the emotional problem and to provide early intervention once the problem is recognized. I subsequently developed the *Care Approach* to mental illness. This approach is intended to provide the first precepts that patients and caregivers should keep in mind and should implement to confront mental illness effectively, especially in its early stages. I also developed the *Help Method* for caregivers and *Heal Technique* for patients in order to empower them in the efficient application of early intervention. The *ABCs of First Aid* were also developed to help patients and caregivers help themselves. A detailed discussion of these approaches is found in Chapters 2, 3, 4, and 5.

Chapters 6 and 7 discuss various coping mechanisms and interventions, such as exposure, desensitization, and anger management, in a step-by-step manner. Each intervention is explored in detail. Chapters 8 to 19 (also referred as the clinical chapters) deal with the common clinical symptoms that patients experience and that caregivers observe in their loved ones. Each of these chapters showcases case scenarios depicting the typical features of a specific symptom, followed by a discussion of the symptoms and associated complications. General information on the various psychiatric disorders presenting with a particular symptom is subsequently provided. Each chapter ends with information on early intervention – a detailed section on the basic do's and don'ts.

The last chapter deals with some of the common psychiatric issues that confront patients and caregivers. Forensic issues such as confidentiality, informed consent, and involuntary hospitalization are explored.

I sincerely hope that this book will provide you or your loved one with simple and yet, essential tools in facing common emotional disorders.

Michael G. Rayel, MD

How To Use This Book

Let me define the terms **patient** and **caregiver** as used in this book. A **patient** refers to any individual suffering from any type of emotional symptom. This definition also applies to individuals who have not yet seen a health care professional. The caregiver refers to an individual who is willing to help and care for the welfare of another including friends, acquaintances, neighbors, personal caretakers, counselors, and spouses or relatives of the emotionally sick person. Temporary caregiver may apply to law enforcement officers who are called to respond during emergencies.

There are several ways of optimizing the use of this book. One way is to leisurely read the whole book from the first to the last chapter, especially if there is no urgency or current need to apply any of its principles and knowledge. A second way is to read appropriate sections of the book for the purpose of helping yourself or a loved one. This option requires you to read Chapters 2 to 7 to learn the basics of first aid to mental illness. The C*are Approach*, *Help Method*, and *Heal Technique*, and *ABCs of First Aid* are concepts that require mastery. The chapters on *basic coping skills* should be examined and learned in detail. After reading these vital chapters, you can proceed to the specific chapter that deals with the emotional problem affecting you or your loved one. You may have to read other appropriate chapters on the presenting symptoms.

While reading a clinical chapter, read the *case scenario*, the *clinical manifestations* of the symptom and its *complications*, the various *emotional disorders* manifesting the symptoms, and then the *early intervention*. From the lists of interventions, choose and apply only the appropriate and relevant measures. If some of these interventions appear to be vague, you may need to reread Chapters 6 to 7 where you will find a detailed discussion of each coping skill.

The third way concerns urgent situations. If there is a need to utilize the early intervention section of a clinical chapter immediately as for example in the case of depression, go directly to that section (the clinical chapters are chapters 8 to 19). Choose from the list of interventions those which are appropriate for that particular situation and apply them. You will still need to read and master the other important chapters when the situation is under control.

The *CARE approach* is reflected in each clinical chapter. For example, in Chapter 8, **C**heck for signs of mental illness corresponds to *how is depression manifested?* **A**nticipate complications corresponds to *what are the complications to anticipate?* **R**emedy with an early intervention refers of course to *early intervention*. And **E**ducate yourself about the illness corresponds to the sections *what are the common illnesses that show depression and early intervention?*

Chapter **1**

Why First Aid to Mental Illness?

Emotional difficulties – a common phenomenon

Emotional and mental difficulties are widespread in the population, and they occur just as frequently as physical disorders. Countless stressors and hassles, such as family conflicts, break-ups between lovers, and problems in the workplace, often cause emotional turbulence. Of course, some individuals handle their emotional difficulties better than others. Individuals who hardly cope experience persistent and worsening symptoms. According to Sharfstein and colleagues (1995), a 1988 US Statistic shows that mental illness, alcohol and drug abuse and their treatment incurred a total cost of about $273.3 billion dollars. About 36% of the total was due to "lost and reduced productivity." Treatment alone constituted 24% of the total. The overall toll exacted from afflicted individuals, caregivers, and society is thus enormous.

Mental illness and stigma

Despite advances in psychiatric research and treatment, mental illness is often misunderstood. Public misconception about mental illness has created unfortunate and inaccurate labels. Many of my patients have remarked that their relatives, who sometimes shame and discredit them, poorly understand their emotional difficulties. Patients have been labeled "lazy" and "weakling," or they have been told to "smarten up," "grow up," and "go to work." Accused of having "weak nerves," of not "pushing hard enough" and of not being "strong enough" to face life's challenges, patients interpret the insults in terms of personal weakness.

Some patients have quietly recognized emotional illness as being "a disgrace," and a "shameful thing" that need not be discussed or expressed openly, even to close relatives. Patients may give their illness a religious meaning. They may think that God is punishing them for their sins and that they deserve to suffer. Or they may believe that "karma" is at work, their current torments stemming from tainted prior lives.

Comparison with physical problems

Physical illnesses, with a few exceptions (such as HIV and venereal disease), carry little or no stigma. People do not hesitate to tell their friends, relatives, neighbors, and co-workers about their flu, allergic reaction to medication, or uncontrolled diabetes. They purchase medications for such conditions at the pharmacy without reservation. However, the situation is quite different for people who suffer from depression, anxiety, or other emotional problems. As stated above, people may hide their symptoms from others if they feel shame or fear criticism. Normally, they do not talk about emotional and behavioral changes, such as crying episodes, mood swings, severe and unrelenting anxiety, obsessive and ruminative thoughts, self-induced vomiting, and hearing voices. Some patients feel ashamed in asking for help. Unlike the case of physical illness, purchasing the medication from the pharmacy represents an unpleasant, strenuous endeavor because they don't want others to "know" about their emotional problems.

Manifestations of mental illness

Unlike physical disorders which have to do with physical changes (such as fever, headache, and nausea), emotional illness is much broader in scope and affects almost all areas of the patient's life. It generally involves a combination of emotional, physical, personality, cognitive, and behavioral changes. Clinical depression is a good example of a mental illness that presents with these changes: e*motional* changes include tearfulness, irritability, loss of interest, and feelings of sadness; *physical* changes include inability to eat, lack of energy, weight loss or gain, lack of sexual drive, and impaired sleep; *personality* changes are manifested through such behavior as easily getting upset or making unusual business decisions; *cognitive* changes include lack of concentration and memory lapses; and *behavioral* changes are shown by agitation and violent tendencies and frequent pacing. The majority, if not all, of patients suffering from mental illness must endure and cope with these modes of change.

Mental illness- a medical disorder

Mental illness, like physical illness, is a medical disorder. Psychiatric research in the past decades has shown its underlying physical mechanisms. Major mental disorders have manifested "chemical imbalance" or neurochemical brain changes (such as those related to serotonin and norepinephrine) found in the brain of clinically depressed individuals. Likewise, abnormality in brain structure is also found in the emotionally ill population, such as the changes observed in schizophrenic patients. Moreover, heredity is prominent in the etiology of the majority of mental illnesses. For example, a significant percentage of manic-depressive patients' first-degree relatives are predisposed to mood disorder. Lastly, changes in hormonal and endocrine functions, as well as in other brain and physical mechanisms, are also involved in the cause of mental illness.

In a way, mental illness can be likened to stroke caused by brain impairment. However, unlike stroke, which paralyzes only one part of the body, mental illness paralyzes the "whole life" of the individual, if left untreated. Fortunately for some, the paralysis is only temporary. Since mental illness is a medical disorder, it should not be considered as a less important form of illness. Like other medical disorders, it should be taken seriously and addressed with respect.

The need for first aid to mental illness

First aid for common physical problems is well established. Preventive measures have been used by people from all walks of life, and are commonly applied to physical problems. Simplified approaches for emergency situations such as cardiopulmonary resuscitation (CPR) have been developed, taught, and applied, saving millions of lives.

Despite the frequency of emotional problems, rapid technological advances, and expansion of psychiatric knowledge, there are currently no simplified approaches to mental illness. The concept of first aid to mental illness is not usually applied. Most existing techniques and approaches are used to teach and guide physicians, therapists and counselors. The psychiatric literature does not provide patients and their caregivers with the necessary tools to manage mental conditions during the initial stages of illness, and to guide them during its crucial stages. More often than not, emotional change will be overlooked. It is not uncommon for symptomatic individuals to get worse, to reach a point of no return – gradually becoming dysfunctional, increasingly unable to perform routine recreational and work activities, and having difficulty in sustaining good relationships with their loved ones. If their situation further deteriorates, they eventually become a threat to themselves and others. Symptomatic individuals "at the end of their rope" have shown self-destructive gestures such as overdosing on pills, slashing their wrists, or deliberately driving the car off the road. Others exhibit violent behavior, threatening the lives of their loved ones. Occasionally, they harbor serious delusions or inappropriate beliefs, such as thoughts that their family is better off in heaven, resulting in the homicide of children or spouses.

Perhaps we can blame the inherent complexity of the emotions for having no simplified approach or first aid to common mental health conditions. Dealing with an emotional difficulty like anger is obviously not the same or as simple as dealing with a superficial cut in a finger. A colleague once stated that because of this complexity, therapists and psychiatrists have developed complex solutions that only the trained and the educated can understand and apply. Hence ordinary individuals, especially those who are ill, and their families and caregivers are left with no tools to utilize when confronted with a serious psychological problem.

When emotional problems start to develop, the majority of individuals and their families are unaware of what is occurring and what to do about it. I have frequently heard from a few perplexed individuals and families statements such as "something is not right" or "he's not the same as he used to be," indicating that they have noticed a significant change in a loved one's life. Despite the awareness, many people do not know what to do when confronted with this type of dilemma, and its complexity bewilders them.

What First Aid to Mental Illness can offer?

In a sense, first aid to mental illness should not be a foreign concept to most people. Many individuals, who have come to my clinic with previous emotional symptoms, have told me that at some point in their lives they got over an emotional hump through their effective use of various coping mechanisms, without the benefit of medication or a visit to a mental health professional. Unknowingly, they had successfully helped themselves through emotional first aid.

This book, First Aid to Mental Illness, attempts to simplify complex approaches to common mental or emotional illnesses. It provides basic information to help symptomatic individuals and their caregivers recognize the presence of emotional difficulty by identifying signs and symptoms present in common mental conditions. This aspect is crucial since many individuals do not know what is occurring when they encounter emotional, behavioral, and other changes. The book also teaches the symptomatic individuals and their relatives what to anticipate if the initial symptoms are allowed to persist and worsen, and appropriate intervention is not provided.

The book also provides basic approaches for early remedy and intervention. If successfully applied, first aid may prevent mental problems from worsening. This portion advocates the *do's and don'ts* of intervention and outlines what an ordinary individual can do under the circumstances. Moreover, the book teaches practical techniques to address a particular issue. Rather than advocate a specific type of psychotherapy or espouse theories of psychology, it addresses the immediate mental problem instead by using simple techniques.

First Aid to Mental Illness illustrates a direct and user-friendly approach for the benefit of patients and caregivers. It teaches a unique approach for each group and empowers individuals during difficult times in their lives.

Chapter **2**

The CARE Approach to First Aid

The **CARE approach** is a simplified way to address proactively emotional and behavioral changes that you or others experience. This approach consists of a four-step process that describes in detail how to recognize a change, what to do once a change is noticed, and how to effectively cope with that change. These easy steps involve recognizing early the unique features of certain mental conditions and their associated complications, facilitating early intervention by using practical tips you can apply immediately, and educating yourself about the illness.

The **CARE approach** involves practical interventions in which you:

>**C**heck for signs of mental illness
>**A**nticipate complications
>**R**emedy with early intervention and
>**E**ducate yourself about the illness.

Check for signs of mental illness

Early recognition of emotional disturbance is the first step. As mentioned earlier, mental illness generally presents with a combination of emotional, psychological, cognitive, physical, and behavioral changes. However, each emotional disorder has unique features and contains clusters of symptoms which distinguish it from other illnesses. Changes found in each disorder vary in acuity, frequency, severity, quality, and duration. Some illnesses may or may not be precipitated by stress. Others indicate changes that happen either suddenly or gradually.

Typically, these changes are not noticed readily, especially in the early stages. Most of the time, you must know yourself or the other person well and know what to look for in order to notice the difference. Several "red flags" however should warn you that an emotional disorder is occurring. It includes self-talk with such statements as: "something is not right," "I don't feel the same," "I feel funny," "he's kind of weird lately," "he's not the same person I know," or "I have to push myself." Another common red flag is an alteration in daily routine and activities. For instance, a very active person slowly becomes apathetic and withdrawn. A housewife, who is usually neat, clean, and meticulous, gradually becomes "sloppy" and unconcerned about her appearance and hygiene. Other red flags include shifts in emotional, perceptual, thought, or physical patterns, such as the urge to cry for no reason; disturbances in energy, sleep, and appetite; suspiciousness; hearing a buzzing sound; and extreme fear or anxiety.

Once you recognize these "red flags," consider taking some practical steps. Check for signs and symptoms to recognize a psychological problem. Signs and symptoms are manifestations of the illness and as such represent a significant shift from some aspects of the person's norm. A typical jolly person, for example, is now constantly crying and getting irritated by minor events. A *sign* is understood in medicine as what is seen or observed in the person, for example tearfulness, restlessness, or talking to oneself. A *symptom* is simply what the sick individual complains about or feels, for example a person expressing anxiety or sadness. In general, signs and symptoms encompass all the changes being experienced. These include experiences of hallucination, irritability, mania, aggression, suspiciousness, talking to oneself, being in a withdrawn state, mutism, physical slowing or psychomotor retardation, and inability to function.

It is important to be alert and observant. Look for any change in patterns. Note the frequency and duration of the changes and determine their severity. How bad do you or your relative really feel? Look for any change in functioning, motivation, daily activities, bodily functions, and dealings with others. Have you or your relative lost interest in doing things? Has the problem affected your normal routine and relationships with others? Next, you need to collect information. Write down emotional problems that occur frequently. List these changes and their frequency. Note the consequences. How has the emotional problem affected you or your sick relative's thinking and judgment? Collecting information is crucial in understanding the whole picture of the emotional difficulty and in presenting an accurate account of the illness to the health care professional who will do the evaluation later.

If possible, you should determine the predominant symptom. Is the presentation mostly depression as manifested by frequent tearfulness, feelings of sadness, or thoughts of death? Is the predominating problem mostly anxiety as shown by constant worrying about trifles, and feeling edgy almost all the time? You must establish the predominant symptom so that you know the type of intervention to apply. Doing this also guides you in what you tell the psychiatrist or mental health professional in the clinic the moment you decide to get help. Do not be upset if you have a hard time determining the major problem since it is the role of the mental health professional to identify the underlying illness. You can, however, help by collecting accurate information and giving that information to the appropriate professional.

Example:
> Mr. U has been feeling "down" for the past six months. He states that there is no reason for him to feel depressed since he has a nice job and a wonderful family. His depression persisted until four weeks ago when he noticed that his sleep became interrupted. He lost weight when his appetite diminished. He could not concentrate at work – to the disappointment of the department head. Eventually, his condition gradually deteriorated to the point where he could not function anymore.

Anticipate complications

Recognition and prevention of complications are the next important steps. Mental conditions, if left untreated or if not addressed early, result in some form of complications. Some complications are typical features of a particular disorder. For example, suicidality is a typical complication of a depressed patient; violence and homelessness are complications of patients suffering from schizophrenia; and starvation and electrolyte imbalance are complications of patients with an eating disorder. Being aware of the possibility of complications should prompt you to attend to the emotional changes right away. Since complications are more difficult to address and treat, preventing their occurrence is crucial.

Occasionally however, the complication may itself be the presenting problem. This holds true for some patients who delay obtaining help for a long time. Without recognizing it, patients gradually become engulfed by the illness and its complications. A few clues indicate that you are now dealing with a complication. First, the signs and symptoms are getting worse or more severe as shown by significant change in emotional and physical health, thought and behavior. For example, you have noticed that your relative has changed from being sad and tearful to becoming extremely suspicious of your every move or severely agitated throughout the day. You may have noticed that the individual has been socially withdrawn, making no attempt to talk to or see any family members or even close friends. You may have observed that poor appetite has resulted in a weight loss of 30 pounds. Secondly, destructive behavior to oneself, others, or property has emerged. You may have noticed lacerations on a person's wrist, or empty bottles next to your son's bed, suggesting an attempted overdose. A neighbor, formerly quiet and wholesome, is now ready to strike anyone he meets. Thirdly, a serious inability to function is revealed. A person who once wanted to go to work enthusiastically, full of energy and motivation, now just prefers to lie down on the couch and do nothing, abandoning usual recreational activities, such as carpentry and handcrafts.

Example:
> *Mr. U could not go to work because his depression became serious. He preferred to lie in bed. He refused to talk to any of his relatives or co-workers. He would not even answer the phone or respond to a knock on his door. Eventually, he began to think that he was better off dead. He was preoccupied with dying and began to plan his death. One day he decided to "end it all."*

Remedy with early intervention

Early remedy or intervention indicates that you address the emotional problem with the goal of preventing further deterioration. Several practical techniques can be learned and applied in dealing with a condition, especially in its early stages. Early remedy can be utilized while awaiting an appointment with a psychiatrist or a mental health worker, or while waiting for a bed in a psychiatric hospital. These interventions can also be used to avoid a relapse after a successful treatment of an acute episode. Some symptomatic individuals who have tried coping techniques have felt relief. Occasionally, patients improve without needing the help of a health care professional.

There are two ways you as a patient or caregiver can perform early intervention successfully. You decide to obtain or provide help, and then you take appropriate action.

Make a decision to obtain or provide help

Once you notice a change and are able to determine the presence of signs and symptoms or possible complications, you should seek help. As a patient, seeking help does not necessarily mean seeing your nearest psychiatrist right away or going to the most convenient emergency room. Seeking help simply means opening communication with close and trusted relatives and friends regarding your concerns and your possible avenues or options. Seeking help may require calling support groups or a 1-800 hot line to seek advice or information. It may mean reading literature and visiting helpful websites to get more information on what you are going through. It also involves having the determination to help yourself by making use of the numerous techniques described in the succeeding chapters. As a caregiver, seeking help may mean contacting the nearest mental health services for information and asking for appropriate guidelines. Meanwhile, you should offer a hand of kindness and accommodate your suffering relative. Making a decision to immediately address the issue is crucial, whatever your course of action.

Indecisiveness delays the effort to get help. Delay can stem from many factors: the stigma of seeing a psychiatrist or a mental health professional, being "too busy," lack of support from family members, or a feeling that hiding the illness is more convenient than showing it. Ask yourself a few questions. Is this something I want to handle myself? Do I want my relatives involved? Do I want to get help right away? You should try to weigh the risks and benefits of indecision, of delay in asking for help, or of handling it yourself. After that, make a decision. Emergency situations, however, such as suicidal and homicidal thoughts and gestures, severe impairment in functioning, and worsening of symptoms, require you to seek professional help as soon as possible.

Take appropriate action

Any important change in a person's emotional state calls for immediate action. The application of appropriate techniques, especially in the early phase of the illness, helps. Basic techniques such as the **HELP** method *for families and caregivers*, and the **HEAL** technique *for patients* as outlined in the next two chapters, respectively can be applied to almost all conditions.

Example:
> *While looking for medications to overdose, Mr. U saw the picture of his smiling grandchildren. In that picture, the note "We love you, grandpa!" was inscribed. He cried and wondered whether it was worth hurting his grandchildren by ending his life. He realized that he was sick and needed help. He phoned his brother and asked for help. His brother, in turn, brought him to the hospital.*

Educate yourself about the illness

Education is basic to dealing with a mental condition. "Knowledge is power," as the saying goes. Information gives you tools to get rid of misconceptions about the illness. Misconceptions especially during times of sickness serve no purpose except to fuel an unstable frame of mind with negativism and to aggravate a volatile situation. Education also gives you more psychological tools to confront and cope with the distressing consequences of the illness and helps lessen shame, blame and guilt. Knowledge about an illness leads to a rational understanding of it, allaying fears lurking in the minds of patients and caregivers and reducing tendencies to attribute the emotional disturbance to personal weakness and past sins. In my practice, I have seen patients and their family members feel relieved when they obtain adequate information about the illness – its mechanisms in the brain, various causes, prognosis, and treatment options.

I once had a patient in my clinic who was seriously distraught. She said that she had been depressed for several months and that she could not function well. She preferred to stay in bed. Her husband could not fully understand what was happening to her and he called her names. He told her to "smarten up." She gradually began to believe what he said. Soon, she began to consider herself as "weak" and blamed herself for the family's woes. When I saw her in the clinic, she told me that she would never get better, that she did not deserve to get better. She felt as if she was a piece of garbage. After my evaluation, I explained to her what I thought her problem was: that she might be suffering from clinical depression, that depression was a form of medical disorder sometimes caused by a genetic predisposition, and that it could be treated with medication. Gradually, she began to change. She stopped crying and listened intently to what I had to say about the illness. Her face began to light up. Before she left my clinic, she told me that she felt better. Her husband came during the next visit. I also educated him about her illness, its causes and treatment. He admitted that some of his behavior had made her worse, and he vowed to try his best to support her.

Patients have experienced more hope and less self-blame after an educational session during visits. Likewise, families and caregivers have been reassured that the situation was not as bad as they originally thought. In short, the more information you have about a particular illness or mental condition, the better you'll be able to cope with it.

It is necessary to learn the possible causes, treatment options and their benefits and side effects, risk factors, and prognosis of the illness. Learn the basic *do's and don'ts* when dealing with mental illness and its consequences. In my experience, patient and caregiver feel more comfortable when they acquire vital information, especially in the early phases of the illness. Try to digest information gradually so that you are not overwhelmed by it. Do not be surprised to learn that similar types of symptoms are found in different mental conditions. For example, depression can occur in major depressive disorder or in schizophrenia patients. Anxiety symptoms, including panic attacks, can occur in various mental disorders. Also, you should realize that a particular psychiatric medication can be used for various kinds of mental conditions. An antidepressant, for instance, can be used not just for depression but also for anxiety disorders such as obsessive-compulsive disorder and panic attacks.

Example:
> *While undergoing hospital treatment, Mr. U began to understand his illness and what he was going through. He began to read about clinical depression and its treatment. He also learned about the manifestations of depression. The more he understood the illness, the more his condition improved. After a few weeks, he was discharged from the hospital.*

Chapter 3

The HELP Method
Early Intervention for Caregivers

Family and caregivers have a major role in the early recognition of an illness and in providing initial interventions to contain its symptoms. Many times, however, families and caregivers of patients do not know their critical role in helping the person in distress. They want to lend a hand but they don't know specifically how they can assist. One caregiver told me that she was aware that her husband exhibited behavioral changes for several months before his hospitalization, but she did not know what she could do under the circumstances. Caregivers try to give their best effort, such as pushing the patient to do a certain activity and giving unsolicited advice, but they are often unaware that their demands and advice are making the person worse. Concerned caregivers and families wonder what they can do to help.

The **HELP** *method* addresses these issues. It is a simplified early intervention that allows families and caregivers to help symptomatic individuals or patients deal effectively with an emotional difficulty. The approach requires you to:

>**H**elp patients through the ABCs of first aid
>**E**mpathize generously
>**L**isten actively and
>**P**revent yourself from getting sick

Case Scenario:

Ms. Q developed "mood swings" for the past few weeks. She was observed to be "too happy" and seemed to be agitated. Her husband thought that something was "not right," since she became hypersexual, very talkative, and never needed any sleep at night. While other household members were asleep in the middle of the night, she was busy cleaning the garage and making phone calls to her neighbors.

Help patients through the ABCs of first aid

To effectively help your sick relative or friend, you must apply simple, practical techniques. These techniques need only the application of common sense and a willingness to open your arms to accommodate the distressed individual. These strategies include the following: 1) Accept the ongoing mental health problem. 2) Assist in addressing issues and in getting a mental health assessment by professional and support services. 3) Be available and supportive. 4) Be alert for any signs of destructive behavior. 5) Clarify safety. 6) Check for worsening of symptoms. 7) Call for help. Please see Chapter 5.

Empathize generously

In dealing with symptomatic individuals in various contexts, showing empathy has a beneficial effect. Constantly learn the art of showing empathy. I have to stress the need to *show* empathy since you may be empathetic but if you don't successfully demonstrate it to the person in pain or distress, this feeling will not have a positive impact on that person. Empathy can only be as good as the actual help it can render to the sick person.

There are a few ways of showing empathy. First, use empathic statements. These are appropriate words, phrases, or statements that you use in reaction to what your relative has to say. Important to empathy is the ability to recognize the patient's feelings or emotional difficulties and to convey your awareness of them effectively to that patient. Some helpful empathic statements include: *you sound very upset . . ., that must have been difficult for you. . . ,*and *sounds like you are feeling a lot of pain inside.*

Example:
> *My mom left us when we were small. She left with another man. My dad ended up drinking a lot every day. When he got home, he'd yell at us, and would call me names. I was left to take care of my sisters and a brother . . .(tears began to flow from her eyes) . . . Nobody bothered to help.*

> You sound very upset that nobody seemed to care.

Secondly, you can show empathy by recognizing the situation of the sick individual and then by letting the person know that you recognize it.

Example:
> *I was only 15 then and yet I had a lot of responsibilities. I had to make sure that my younger brother and sisters went to school. I had to work at McDonald's to make sure that there was food on the table. Meanwhile, my dad just continued to drink.*
>
> It was a difficult moment for you.

Another powerful way of conveying your empathy is through the use of pauses or silence. This gesture is applied "in response" to your relative's expression of distress, emotion or concern. If used properly, it may encourage the individual to open up and talk about the emotional difficulty and its circumstances.

Example:
> *One night while everyone was asleep, my dad came home drunk. He went to his room and yelled for coffee. After I gave him the coffee, he held my hand so tight that I couldn't move. He pushed me down to his bed . . .(pause) . . . then . . .* (her eyes became slightly moist with tears) . . .
>
> Pause before answering or asking a question.

Offering a tissue during a tense and tearful episode is an empathic gesture that may mean a lot to these distressed individuals. If you are a close relative or a spouse, a hug or a rub on the back may provide comfort and warmth.

Listen actively

Listening in a manner that shows your interest in the individual's concerns and issues is a useful skill to develop. Frequent eye contact and remarks acknowledging the person's predicament such as *I see, it's too bad,* and *I know* are constructive ways of encouraging the distressed individual to talk. Facilitate the person's story and description of mental anguish through proper gestures such as head nodding. Brief comments, such as *oh my, yeah,* and *uh oh,* encourage the person to communicate highly charged emotions. The sick individual is likely to appreciate your gesture, and the process may strengthen the relationship you have established.

You can usually allow your sick relative to talk "freely" for a significant period. This "free talk" phase allows your relative to talk spontaneously about preoccupations and concerns. Through free talk, your relative is able to talk about preoccupations or issues that matter such as a job loss that has resulted in emotional difficulties, or vice versa. Moreover, letting your sick relative talk freely enhances your relationship. It builds an alliance by giving the person a feeling of importance through an unrestricted expression of one's problems, concerns, and emotion.

Free talk can be facilitated by the use of open-ended questions. In daily conversation, we tend to use open-ended questions liberally. Some phrases that facilitate free talk are: *tell me about . . . , what. . ? , how . . ?* , among others. Refrain from *why* questions because very often the patients will not know the answer and it places them in a defensive mode.

Allow persons to talk about anything regularly at certain times. How often and how long will you let the sick person talk freely? Your comfort level is the key. If you feel comfortable letting your relative talk freely for thirty minutes a day, then by all means do so. On the other hand, do not allow yourself to be overwhelmed by allowing the patient to talk *constantly*, giving you no time to fulfill your commitments and responsibilities, or to rest for a while.

Example:
    What made you see a psychiatrist?

I don't really know what happened. But I just felt I was superwoman. I was very energetic despite not sleeping well. I had the feeling that I could do anything. I was in fact overconfident in making business deals and in meeting new faces. It all started when my supervisor was giving me a hard time. He even threatened to fire me.

That's too bad. What happened then?

It happened two months ago. I noticed some accounting errors and I made him aware of it. He got so upset. He blamed me for everything. He told me I'm no good and all that stuff.

I see.

Prevent yourself from getting sick

You cannot effectively help your distressed relative or family member if you do not maintain your own mental and emotional health. Many families and caregivers, however, get sick after weeks or months of handling the difficulty associated with the illness. If you are not careful, the stress of caregiving will take its toll. It is unfortunate if a caregiver becomes as sick as or possibly sicker than the symptomatic individual.

The rule of thumb in assisting a symptomatic individual is: *Keep yourself healthy during the whole process.* This can be achieved by immersing yourself in various positive and uplifting activities that represent physical, nutritional, spiritual, social, and mental needs such as regular exercise, balanced diet, adequate sleep, attending church, visiting friends, and playing scrabble with neighbors. *Learn various coping mechanisms and new skills and activities.* Practical ways to relax and relieve tension, to deal with anger, and to communicate properly, can go a long way in keeping you ahead of the illness. The details of these skills are discussed in Chapters 6 and 7. *Join a support group or obtain support from close and trusted friends and family members.* The quality of reassurance and support you get from others determines your quality of life and emotional health. Obtaining help from relatives, friends, community, church, and community agencies has a positive impact on the help you provide to your distressed relative.

*Some portions of this chapter were adapted from the book: Successful Preparation For the Psychiatry Oral Exam by Michael G. Rayel, MD

Chapter **4**

The HEAL Technique
Early Intervention for Patients

Just like the caregivers, patients have expressed concerns that they lack know-how in recognizing emotional changes and in confronting emotional difficulties in their early stages. Even if they sense that "something is wrong," they often have no idea about what might really be happening. Also, in most cases, patients have no idea what to do. They are ashamed to share their predicament with colleagues at work, friends or even family. Even those they confide in are usually unsure about how to help. Consequently, patients feel lost and alone as they try to grapple with an unchartered emotional territory. Unnecessary delay occurs. Before they realize it, their minimal symptoms have reached a critical point, representing a grave stage of the illness.

The **HEAL** *technique* is intended to fill this void. The technique simplifies the process of early intervention to aid you when you become emotionally ill. It tells you what to do and how to help yourself once you notice a change. It guides you to take basic steps to prevent the worsening of the illness by addressing the relevant issues. The technique encourages you to learn coping mechanisms to help you handle your crisis. Timely application of these techniques is a must. The **HEAL** techniques strongly recommend you to:

Help yourself through ABCs of first aid
Encourage yourself
Address the issues and
Learn to cope

Case Scenario:

> *Mr. S complained of severe anxiety for many years. Since childhood, he had experienced "butterflies" in his stomach. Recently, he had become more anxious after he lost his job. He would worry excessively about anything, even minor things. He could not concentrate on his job. He felt tense as if always on edge. At night, he could hardly sleep.*

Help yourself through ABCs of first aid

This technique offers a practical approach to assist in confronting your emotional issue. This approach does not require an understanding of psychological theories and intensive training. Only your determination to help yourself is necessary as you clear your emotional hurdle. These approaches include the following: 1) Accept the ongoing mental health problem. 2) Be alert for signs of destructive thoughts and behavior. 3) Check for worsening of symptoms. 4) Call for help. A detailed discussion is found in Chapter 5.

Example:
> *Mr. S acknowledged that his symptoms are out of the ordinary. He further concluded that his anxiety had become worse and had affected his work efficiency. He realized that he needed treatment. Mr. S sought advice from close friends and relatives. After he was given options, he decided to check the Yellow Pages looking for a physician's clinic. He subsequently booked an appointment to see a psychiatrist.*

Encourage yourself

Encouraging yourself, especially at the early stages of the illness, is beneficial for the long haul. Keeping yourself encouraged is necessary to face emotional obstacles. You must stay positive and energetic as you travel along life's difficult course. You can keep yourself encouraged by immersing yourself in positive and worthwhile endeavors. Read positive literature daily such as religious articles, self-help or how-to books, and enthusiastic quotes. Your speech must also be positive especially when you talk to yourself. Avoid self-blame, self-doubt, and self-criticism. Feed your mind with refreshing and inspiring thoughts. Try to associate with people who are able to give heartening words. Watch inspiring movies and TV shows. Avoid negativism. You cannot afford to harbor negative thoughts at this point in time. Although your illness can trigger self-criticism and self-blame, always try to maintain a positive outlook.

Meanwhile, discouragement is an indication of worse things to come. Do not allow discouragement to set foot in your emotional household since it will fuel more negative feelings. This is not the time to be discouraged and it is not the time to associate yourself with people who shower harsh words and who spread negative attitudes.

Example:
> *Mr. S began to read books on mental health, particularly on anxiety disorders. He also liked reading uplifting and inspiring books and magazines. He began to talk to people who went through the same illness and who successfully recovered.*

Address the issues

Address the issues, whether familial, personal, or interpersonal, that trigger the symptoms and make your emotional health worse. In addressing some personal and interpersonal issues, make use of the various coping mechanisms discussed in Chapters 6 and 7 such as anger management, assertiveness techniques, and problem-solving strategies. In solving problems, for instance, some basic steps can help. First, identify the root cause or precipitant of the problem. You may be depressed because of a failing marriage. You then identify your marriage as an area needing intervention. You may have multiple problems. Still, it is important to identify them and prioritize them according to their degree of importance. Secondly, seek solutions and explore options. If your marriage has been "on the rocks" for several months, pursue options such as marriage counseling, divorce, separation, or settlement through a family mediator. Thirdly, consider the risk and benefits of each option. You may both realize, for example, that you still love each other and that making the marriage work and giving yourselves a chance to iron out wrinkles in the relationship would be beneficial. The risk, however, of this choice includes the possibility of more arguments and conflict within the marriage. Fourthly, make a choice and act. Both of you, for instance, might decide to consider marriage counseling as the best option. You finally may see a marriage counselor to resolve issues and concerns.

The key is to meet the problem head-on as early as possible. Denying the existence of the problem or refusing to address it in a timely fashion can result in undesirable long-term effects.

Example:
> *After the initial visit with the psychiatrist, Mr. S felt confident that help was within reach. He was put on medications. He also underwent talk therapy for a few weeks. After recovering from the illness, he developed the strength to give himself another chance in the workforce. He contacted friends and co-workers about available positions. He also submitted his resume to several companies.*

Learn to cope

Coping mechanisms, such as breathing exercises, activity scheduling, and progressive muscle relaxation can make you feel better when under stress and may even regenerate you. Moreover, coping mechanisms may serve as "treatment" especially when practiced regularly, relieving you of needless pressure and gnawing symptoms. As mentioned before, these coping skills should be used to reduce the symptoms especially while awaiting an appointment with a mental health professional. They can be applied to prevent the deterioration of a persistent condition. There are some patients who, after regular application and utilization of coping skills, realize that they can go back to their usual selves even without the benefit of medications or therapy sessions. A detailed discussion on coping skills is found in the next chapter.

Example:
> *Mr. S was taught several coping mechanisms during his visits with the psychiatrist. He practiced breathing exercises and progressive muscle relaxation on a daily basis. He organized his daily schedule to accommodate recreational activities such as taking walks, gardening, and knitting. He also pursued his spiritual interests.*

Chapter 5

ABCs of First Aid

The **ABCs** are major components of the HELP and HEAL approaches and are crucial strategies for early intervention especially in attempting to help others or yourself. They involve acknowledging the illness and being extremely alert to worsening condition and developing destructive thoughts and behavior. They require being available and able to assist in getting timely assessment. Moreover, they demand calling for help especially if a safety issue is a major concern.

Case Scenario:

Ms. Q developed "mood swings" for the past few weeks. She was observed to be "too happy" and seemed to be agitated. Her husband thought that something was "not right," since she became hypersexual, very talkative, and never needed any sleep at night. While other household members were asleep in the middle of the night, she was busy cleaning the garage and making phone calls to her neighbors.

Accept the ongoing mental health problem

Accepting that there is a problem is the first essential step. Denying the presence and the gravity of the situation will not stand you or the symptomatic individual in good stead. Blaming others will prevent you and the sick person from solving the problem. *Normalizing* the illness, that is, considering the symptoms as part of a normal process, detracts from seeking appropriate treatment. The rule of thumb is to accept the ongoing emotional difficulty and then cope with it.

Example:
> *Ms. Q's husband concluded that Ms. Q possibly had an emotional problem. He accepted the current difficulties as possibly caused by a mental illness and decided to deal with it appropriately.*

Assist in addressing issues and in getting a mental health assessment by professional and support services

Symptomatic individuals, who are very distressed and unable to think clearly, need assistance in asking for help and in scheduling an appointment with a mental health professional. Occasionally, the individual's poor judgment brought on by the illness impedes efforts to seek help. Likewise, the sick person's lack of understanding about his/her mental condition works against obtaining necessary treatment. Your role as a caregiver is to make a genuine attempt to seek help and advice from health professionals about the most appropriate plan of action.

Helping patients address problems is another way of providing assistance. Many affected individuals have suffered from various kinds of stressors. Some patients have been experiencing serious conflicts with their spouses. You may serve as a mediator between the conflicting couple and assist them with solutions. A patient may have just lost a job or may have recently been charged with a crime. In helping unemployed persons, you can show the proper way to write a resume or offer to mail applications on their behalf. For someone charged with a crime, you can advise the distressed person to acquire the services of a good lawyer in order to gain a better understanding of the legal situation. Remember that obtaining accurate information can help allay fear and anxiety.

Example:
> *Ms. Q's husband decided to call the nearest mental health center. He discussed his wife's emotional problems with a counselor and acquired some understanding about the changes in her life. He immediately made an appointment for her to see the psychiatrist.*

> *Ms. Q's illness was precipitated by a "conflict" with her supervisor at work. She felt that because she made an accounting mistake, she would be fired. Her husband decided to clarify the issue with her supervisor. He learned that there was simply a misunderstanding and that there was no definite strain in the relationship. Her supervisor decided to visit her to "patch things up."*

Be available and supportive

Your availability and support as a caregiver is much needed during this period of emotional turmoil. Unnecessary blaming and "guilt tripping" should stop and arguments should be avoided since they just make matters worse. Being supportive does not mean that you always support the sick person's choices or actions, including those with potential negative consequences. Being supportive simply means that you support anything that is beneficial for the sick person.

Availability does not mean being there 24 hours a day, but it does require that you be there when you are needed the most. It also means being with the person regularly and for as long as necessary. For instance, I have a patient whose mother visits her everyday for at least one hour to talk about her concerns and issues. During this time, the mother also helps with the chores.

Example:
> *Ms. Q's husband decided to ask for a leave from work to be at her side during this period of immense emotional difficulty. He would also talk to her and listen to her complaints and concerns.*

Be alert for any signs of destructive behavior

Suicidal and homicidal gestures as manifested by wrist slashing, overdosing on drugs, and assaultive and aggressive behavior are signs of a serious illness. Be aware that these are emergency situations which most likely require psychiatric hospitalization. As a caregiver, you should look for any wounds or marks on the patient's neck or wrist. Also, watch out for more *subtle* signs such as empty bottles next to the person's bed, a "lost" prescription, frequent accidents, planning to buy a rope, and changing one's will.

As a patient, watch out for any change, especially when you begin to feel "different" as you experience unusual thoughts or engage in uncommon behavior patterns. You may start to feel that death is a more "worthwhile option" than living. You may think that you and your family members are "better off in heaven" than in this world. You easily "snap" over minor things and get agitated and violent for no reason. When these types of feelings

ABCs of First Aid

and thoughts appear, be aware that they are abnormal patterns that need to be addressed soon by a mental health professional or your family doctor. There is no need to ask further why it is happening. You just need to act right away.

Example:
> Ms. Q's husband closely monitored her demeanor and behavior for a few days. He observed that Ms. Q would drive the car very fast and much above the speed limit in their neighborhood. He also learned that Ms. Q had withdrawn $25,000 from their bank account and spent it all on a one-day shopping spree. A week ago, she suddenly "disappeared" for a few days, driving aimlessly on the highway.

Clarify safety

Monitor any change in the person's demeanor. Observe the sick person closely. Do not hesitate to ask the individual, especially one with depression, psychosis, anxiety, substance abuse, or a combination of problems, about any suicidal or homicidal thoughts. You will not drive the sick person to suicide or homicide by doing so. When you clarify safety, do so in a subtle way. You may ask, for example, if your sick relative has *thoughts that life is not worth living anymore*. Or alternatively, you may ask if he or she is *better off dead*. If you know the person well and you've been honest with each other in the past, you may directly ask the question such as: *are you suicidal?* Or *have you had thoughts about ending your life?* Before you ask these direct questions, prepare the way by first allowing the patient to express emotions, to talk about concerns, and to feel comfortable and secure. Then try to clarify safety.

Example:
> Ms. Q's husband wondered whether she had thought about hurting herself or others. He therefore asked her whether she ever preferred to die rather than to live. When she said no, he inquired if she considered hitting people when they get on her nerves.

Check for worsening of symptoms

As a caregiver, monitor your sick relative's presentation. Observe if there is further deterioration of the person as shown by significant weight loss, disheveled appearance, inability to function, bizarre behavior, severe distress, and presence of suicidal and homicidal gestures. Verify whether the patient has progressively isolated himself/herself from relatives, close friends, and the outside world.

As a patient, any delay in seeking help is harmful to your mental health. Mental illness, if left untreated, becomes unmanageable. Gradually, you become aware that the symptoms have increased in intensity. You have become, for instance, more anxious and depressed. Perhaps your sleep has been reduced, and the impairment in your functioning has gone from bad to worse. Be alert and observant and constantly monitor your emotional status. Do not allow the emotional problem to arrive at a critical stage where help may be out of reach.

Example:
> Ms. Q's husband observed her to be hyperactive. She would not stay at home especially at night. She frequented bars and had sexual liaisons with several acquaintances in one night. One day while driving the car, she hit a truck resulting in extensive damage to her car. Luckily she came out unharmed. The next day, she made deals with the top businessmen in town. She thought that in order for them to succeed, she had to help them out.

Call for help

As a caregiver, ask for help if necessary. Call the emergency room of a nearby hospital if emergency situations, such as suicidal and homicidal gestures, are evident. Inquire about what to do if the sick person refuses to be brought to the hospital. Call the 1-800 hotlines for information and advice regarding the appropriate approach to a sick person in need of immediate assistance. You might call law enforcement agencies, especially if violence or homicidal gestures are involved. With the sick person's health deteriorating, call a nearby medical clinic for help.

As a patient, make sure that you ask for help before the illness gets out of hand. Any further delay will make the illness more difficult to treat. Also, the illness at its worst will render you unaware of the need to seek help, since at this stage, you may already have a profound lack of understanding about the situation. Do not hesitate to approach a mental health clinic or seek the help of community agencies. Check the phonebook for support groups and organizations, and attempt to connect with them. Talk to your close friends and relatives about your predicament and ask if they can assist you. Go to the emergency room if you experience a worsening of your symptoms and if you have thoughts of death.

Example:
> Her husband was extremely bothered by her emotional and behavioral changes. He decided to talk to their parish priest for

advice. The priest suggested calling the emergency room in the nearby town.

Chapter **6**

Basic Coping Skills to Help Deal with Mental Illness 1

Coping skills have a significant role to play in prevention, in reducing the signs and symptoms, in effectively confronting the issues, and in minimizing the impact of the illness. When used appropriately and promptly, both patients and caregivers can benefit from these strategies. For example, a male patient learns assertiveness techniques and problem-solving skills to help him deal with everyday demands while a mother practices anger management when dealing with an intoxicated, alcoholic son. Below, you will find the commonly recognized coping mechanisms and their simplified and modified versions.

Breathing Exercises

Breathing exercises consist of a slow cycle of inhalation through the nose and exhalation through the mouth with the intention of achieving relaxation. This is one of the most "portable" relaxation exercises because you can do the technique at any time and place. For example, you can perform it in a restaurant if you start to feel anxious being around people. This exercise is indicated for stress, anxiety, and anger reduction. Optimal relaxation is achieved if this exercise is done in combination with other exercises noted below such as visualization or progressive muscle relaxation. The process includes the following:

> A. Sit or lie down comfortably. (the latter is preferable if the exercise is done in private). To prevent dizziness, avoid this exercise while walking or standing up.
> B. Close your eyes. (You don't have to close your eyes in a public place such as a restaurant.)
> C. Begin a cycle of slow inhalation through the nose and slow exhalation through the mouth with a pause in between. Do this exercise by counting between three to five seconds in each phase.
> D. Do the routine for five to ten minutes or until you feel relaxed.
> E. Do the exercise regularly such as twice a day or at your most stressful time during the day.

Progressive Muscle Relaxation

Progressive muscle relaxation, indicated for anxiety, phobia, stress, and anger, is achieved through a cycle of tensing and then releasing a group of muscles throughout your body. Start with the muscle groups of the lower extremities such as the toes, feet, calf, and thighs. Then you proceed to the hip and buttocks and gradually go up to the abdominal area. Next, tense and relax your upper extremities such as your fingers, hands, forearms, and arms. Proceed to tense and relax the chest, back and shoulder areas, then the neck region, and eventually, the facial area. You can reverse the order of muscle relaxation – from upper extremities down to the toes, in your next session. The key is to be able to tense and relax all muscle groups thoroughly.

Tensing of each muscle group can last several seconds. You can do this exercise for about fifteen to twenty minutes while sitting or lying down. You can try it longer if you still experience tension in your body, until you achieve relaxation. You can do muscle relaxation in your office or bedroom.

Visualization

Visualization is a type of mental exercise that puts you into a different reality. It can put you in almost any place, and induce a comfortable and refreshing state. Achieving calmness and tranquility follows after a few minutes of performing this mental exercise. Visualization can be used in a variety of situations including anxiety, extreme tension, stress, and anger.

There are three steps to follow in this exercise. First, put yourself in a relaxed state through breathing exercises or progressive muscle relaxation or a combination of both. Other patients have tried physical exercise in combination with muscle relaxation or breathing exercise to achieve a similar result. Secondly, with your eyes closed, visualize yourself in a very comfortable, relaxing, and enjoyable place. For example, picture yourself walking on the shores of sunny Florida. Remember that you should put yourself in a place where *you* feel comfortable and relaxed. It can be anywhere – in the woods, near rivers, ponds, mountains, ski trails, or even on the balcony of your house. Thirdly, experience the place using all your five senses. For example, while walking on the sunny beach, you enjoy the sight of children playing in the sand. You feel the warm air gently touching your body and face. You can hear the waves as they collide with the rocky coastline. Do this exercise for several minutes until you achieve full relaxation.

Desensitization and Exposure Technique

Joseph Wolpe originally developed a technique known as systematic desensitization. It is a type of coping and therapeutic technique that involves gradual and imaginary exposure to the anxiety-provoking events or situations along with relaxation-inducing activities such as progressive muscle relaxation. It consists of several steps and is known to be effective in dealing with phobia or fear associated with certain situations. Below, you will find a modified technique that combines virtual and actual exposure along with relaxation phase.

A. Create hierarchy of the anxiety-provoking event

Exposure to an anxiety-provoking event has always been part of the intervention in dealing with a specific anxiety-provoking stimulus. Although some individuals feel comfortable with sudden exposure to the event as part of treatment, the majority of my patients prefer a gradual experience. With regard to the latter, it is necessary to establish a graduated list of stimuli or events, ranging from the least to the most anxiety-provoking and feared events. The exposure can be done in two ways: The first way is through virtual exposure. This type of exposure involves a) visualizing the fear-inducing stimuli, b) watching a video of the stimuli, or c) looking at (or touching) a picture of the feared stimuli. For effective results, these three types of virtual exposure can be combined. The second method involves actual exposure. This type of exposure is done in reality – there is actual contact with the stimuli in question.

For example, a male patient, who has a phobia about cockroaches resulting in severe distress and impairment in functioning, may create a list that will appear as:

> **Virtual exposure**: he visualizes that 1) a kitchen cabinet contains a bottle that has two cockroaches inside; 2) he is opening the cabinet;

3) he is looking at the cockroaches inside the bottle from afar; 4) he is looking at the cockroaches about a foot away; 5) cockroaches are getting out of the bottle; 6) cockroaches are crawling on the person's feet.

Actual exposure: 1) he is looking at the kitchen cabinet with actual cockroaches inside the bottle; 2) he is opening the kitchen cabinet; 3) he is looking at the cockroaches inside the bottle from afar; 4) he is looking at the cockroaches inside the bottle from about a foot away; 5) he is touching the bottle with cockroaches inside; 6) the cockroaches are let out of the bottle while the person is standing close by.

B. Relaxation phase

This is a significant part of the behavioral intervention. The patient induces relaxation in ten to twenty minutes through a variety of techniques including breathing exercises and progressive muscle relaxation. The patient may combine these exercises to achieve a calm and tranquil state.

C. Pleasant imagery

Once relaxation is achieved, the patient should now visualize being in a comfortable and refreshing place. This imagery is highly individualized and reflects your personal preference. You use all senses to create a total experience of the place. For example, you visualize yourself walking along the shores of a white sandy beach. You hear the waves as they approach the shore while you watch the seagulls soar in the bright blue sky. You feel warmth as the sunlight meets your tanned skin, you stoop to feel the fine grains of sand, and you savor the ocean smells.

D. Virtual exposure to anxiety-provoking event

While in a relaxed state, visualize yourself exposed to the anxiety-provoking stimulus, starting with the first or least anxiety-provoking stimulus or event in the hierarchy. For example, you visualize the kitchen cabinet with two cockroaches inside a bottle. Stay exposed for several seconds. If you don't experience any distress or discomfort with that specific stimulus, proceed to the next one. You now, for instance, visualize opening the cabinet with cockroaches. When you develop anxiety to a certain stimulus or event, try to stay with this particular event as long as you can to help yourself adapt. However, you may decide to stop and go back to pleasant imagery if the event induces an overwhelming experience.

E. Back to pleasant imagery

Once anxiety becomes distressful or overwhelming, visualize the pleasant scenery and stay there for several seconds until you feel relaxed.

F. Repetitive virtual exposure until mastery

Repeat your virtual exposure to a particular event until you are quite comfortable. For instance, you visualize repetitively the opening of the kitchen cabinet. Gradually move up the hierarchy until you have fully mastered the events in the list. You know that you have achieved mastery if you can think about the stimuli or events without inducing anxiety or discomfort.

G. Actual exposure

Proceed with the hierarchy requiring actual exposure to the stimuli or events. Start with the easy or least fear-inducing stimulus and then progress slowly. You may, for instance, start with just looking at the kitchen cabinet with cockroaches inside.

H. Withdraw to a comfortable state if unable to tolerate the exposure

Each time a distress or discomfort is induced by a specific event, visualize pleasant imagery, and engage in breathing exercises or progressive muscle relaxation or a combination of these three. You may perform these relaxation exercises repeatedly.

I. Repetitive actual exposure until mastery

Expose yourself gradually to the next stage on the list. Continue the process until you have fully covered the hierarchy on the list and have achieved mastery. By this time, any form of exposure to the anxiety-inducing event, such as the cockroach, will not elicit anxiety or distress anymore.

Exposure

This technique is related to the desensitization and exposure technique described above. The only difference is that you don't have to induce relaxation through relaxation and visualization techniques. Exposure is indicated for phobic disorders and feelings of dread of certain situations or events (such as fear of contamination). It can be done abruptly or gradually. Abrupt exposure is effective, but it may elicit an overwhelming experience of dread and fear in the early phase. An individual who is scared of dogs, for instance, is told to massage the head of a puppy. The initial phase is anxiety provoking, but once the person realizes that it is actually safe to hold a puppy, then the overpowering emotions slowly subside. Abrupt exposure is not recommended for everyone.

Gradual exposure is more subtle than the abrupt method because overwhelming emotions are avoided. This technique can be very effective in dealing with common fears and phobias. The step-by-step process is provided below.

Establish hierarchy

Just like in the previous technique, you need to create a hierarchy of stimuli or events, ranging from the least to the most anxiety-provoking. You may start the exposure with virtual and then go to actual.

Imaginary or virtual exposure

This phase involves gradual exposure to the anxiety-provoking stimuli or events through visualization. You start with the easiest and gradually go to the most difficult or anxiety-provoking event. If a stimulus causes substantial distress, stop the exercise temporarily. After a period of rest (such as a few minutes), restart the exercise where you left off and continue the process.

Actual exposure

Actual exposure to the stimuli is the final goal of this exercise. At the end, you should be able to "embrace" the object of dread.

Gradual and repetitive exposure until mastery

Repetitive exposure should result in mastery. It may take weeks or months, for some even years, but eventually the exercise will pay off.

Example:
> A patient who fears dogs can do the following exercises: First, use virtual exposure by looking at a picture of a dog from a distance, then looking at the picture more closely. Followed this by actually touching the dog in the picture, and finally "embracing" the picture of the dog for at least ten minutes. Secondly, use actual exposure by looking at the dog from a distance, then looking at the dog from about one foot away, followed by stroking the dog's back for a few

seconds, then massaging the dog's back for several minutes, and finally embracing the dog.

Thought Restructuring

Thought restructuring refers to the use of strategies to deal with inappropriate or maladaptive thoughts that cause distress and emotional disturbance. These inappropriate thoughts include memories of painful and traumatic experiences in the past, ruminative thoughts about current concerns, and the so-called "automatic" shoulds and musts as noted by cognitive-behavioral therapists. Thought restructuring requires you to develop an alternative more appropriate thought process. This technique is indicated for any type of conditions, such as depression, anger, obsession, and anxiety.

Identify inappropriate thoughts

Inappropriate thoughts are usually negative and unproductive thoughts that create negative changes in your emotions. These thoughts make you emotionally turbulent and elicit a spectrum of emotion including hostility, anger, anxiety, and depression. Since they are usually negative, they lower self-confidence and diminish your self-respect. Such thoughts include those thoughts labeled "cognitive distortions" by cognitive behavioral therapists, such as generalizations (e.g. *"All cars made by General Motors are excellent because the Cavalier I bought last year is running well."*), jumping to conclusions (e.g. *"She didn't smile at me this morning. I believe that she hates me"*), and all or none thinking (e.g. *"I'm not really a good student because I made a few mistakes in the exam."*).

Inappropriate thoughts can encompass a lot more than cognitive distortions. They include thoughts about bad experiences in the past, serious concerns of the present, intrusive and recurrent thoughts, and worry about the future. Examples include wrongs done in the past by your ex-husband, slights received from your co-workers, and the rape you experienced as a teenager. Intrusive thoughts are unwanted and unacceptable thoughts that intrude regularly into your awareness despite your attempts to get rid of them. These might include murderous or blasphemous thoughts.

Try to be observant. List those thoughts that give you distress and keep you awake at night. Be aware of those thoughts that preoccupy you constantly and disturb your peace of mind.

Interventions

Once you realize that you harbor inappropriate thoughts, make a conscious effort to deal with them through the following techniques. First, attempt to practice replacement, that is, replacing the inappropriate thought with a completely different thought. For example, instead of thinking about your abusive relationships in the past, focus your mind on your career goals. Second, try diversion. Use both physical and psychosocial components (as shown below). Third, give yourself a time-out from the negative thoughts. For example, you decide to stop the negative rumination for several hours per day. You could also *delay* its onslaught by telling yourself, "I'll think about it later in the afternoon." The details of diversion and time-out are described more fully in the next sections. Fourth, practice positive self-talk frequently. Talk to yourself repetitively about the positive outcome and expectations. For example, you may tell yourself, "I'm focusing on my goals and will pursue them relentlessly." Fifth, signal yourself to stop each time an inappropriate thought occurs. For instance, every time your mind starts to drift to negative ruminations or intrusive thoughts, tell yourself *enough of this!* Then, try diversion or thought replacement. Sixth, analyze the benefits or disadvantages of harboring those inappropriate thoughts. Consider their consequences to your emotional and physical health, and to your whole life. And seventh, make a decision to end their control on your life.

Diversion

Diversion is a coping technique that keeps you away from disturbing emotions and distressing thoughts. This technique requires effort because it is often difficult to divert your mind from negative ruminations. However, if you wish to feel better, then you must use certain techniques. Stop distressing thoughts by doing something abrupt or noticeable, such as seeing a stop signal in your mind, suddenly changing your body position, or slapping your wrist.

Mental diversion

Mental diversion involves changing focus or simply replacing distressful thoughts when undergoing a difficult moment or emotional turmoil. A few techniques can be tried. First, replace the disturbing thoughts with pleasant, positive, or neutral thoughts. Each time the disturbing thought starts to emerge, signal yourself to stop mentally. A stop signal can take various forms such as an image of a pen dropping to the floor, or an image of a stopwatch, and an image of a blinking red light. After creating the stop signal, immediately start having a completely different thought. If, for instance, you begin to ruminate about what your brother did to hurt you, you stop the train of thought by suddenly examining the details of your cell phone or the flower vase in your office. Secondly, focus solely on pleasant or neutral thoughts. Here, you don't allow the negative rumination to start or set in.

You just engross your mind with a neutral or pleasant thought, such as focusing on your business goals for the next two months. This technique is challenging since many patients slip back to negative rumination despite effort. But if you practice this technique constantly, then your efforts will be rewarded. Thirdly, you can replace your negative brooding with thoughts about solutions to your problems. In this technique, you not only replace the thought, but also find ways to address your concerns and burdens. Actively seek answers and solutions.

Physical diversion

Physical diversion involves physical activity to divert your mind from distressing thoughts and your body from disturbing emotions. One way to divert is to keep yourself busy the whole day. Being busy does not give you the time and luxury of negative rumination. Secondly, doing physical exercise serves the same purpose because you tend to focus on your body and respiration rather than on the distressing thoughts. Moreover, the process itself releases a lot of tension from your muscles resulting in a more relaxed state. Thirdly, recreational and other productive activities provide a sense of relief due to the enjoyment you feel during and after the process. You tend to focus on the pleasurable and enjoyable moment rather than on the distressing thoughts. The sense of relief results in a sense of accomplishment.

Social diversion

This type of diversion involves social activities such as visiting friends and relatives, attending social gatherings and functions, involving oneself in community activities, volunteering one's services, or being active in organizations.

Chapter **7**

Basic Coping Skills to Help Deal with Mental Illness 2

Problem-solving Strategies

This technique is a practical way of confronting an ongoing issue. Problems arise everyday and if left unaddressed, they become more complex and difficult, sometimes leading to new problems.

Identify the problems

The first step is to identify the problem, the root cause of the current difficulty. If you address only the consequences rather than the underlying problem, then most likely you will fail. For instance, if you try to address an ongoing marital difficulty without addressing the root cause, such as the gambling of the spouse, the marital problems will persist if the treatment of gambling is not included in the overall therapeutic intervention.

Offer realistic solutions

Once the problem is identified, try to brainstorm for possible solutions. Consider the most realistic one with reference to both short and long-term benefits. Involve your spouse if the solution calls for collaboration and make sure that both parties agree with the plan. Think about the cost and accessibility of the solution.

Weigh the advantages and disadvantages of each alternative

Weigh the risks and benefits of each solution. Write down every point so that you won't miss any crucial ideas. Think hard and don't rush. Ask for advice from credible sources. Eliminate irrelevant ideas from your list. Evaluate the solutions in terms of their overall benefit.

Make a choice and apply

Choose the best alternative among the choices, and then act. Don't delay your action. Be decisive.

Accept the consequences

Be prepared for the consequences. Of course, you expect the best outcome since you have used your best judgment during the deliberation process. But if the consequences are not what you expect, you have to accept the results. But at the same time, you can reconsider your decision and perhaps make another choice.

Assertiveness Technique

Assertiveness technique consists of a variety of strategies to effectively express yourself (your wants, opinion, ideas, inquiries, likes and dislikes) in a diplomatic way without hurting the feelings of others. It involves three basic techniques. First, introduce a pleasant or conducive atmosphere; second, say what you want in a polite manner; and third, be firm.

Introduce a pleasant or conducive atmosphere

Before you say anything, you should create the context in which the other person can listen to what you have to say. Some authors call this technique "disarming." This term is somewhat inaccurate because many individuals are not necessarily "armed" when they deal with you. In fact, many of them are receptive to what you have to say if you say it in a proper way. You establish a pleasant atmosphere by: a) partially agreeing to what the other person says, b) appreciating something about the person, c) avoiding arguments even when you completely disagree, d) speaking in an appropriate tone, and e) talking about something in common, such as family.

Say what you want in a polite manner

After you have created a pleasant conversational atmosphere, speak in a polite and diplomatic way. Some authors and therapists recommend the use of *I* rather than of *you* when expressing your feelings so as to avoid appearing in an accusatory mode. For example: *I'm upset that I was made to feel dumb last night* is a better expression than *you made me feel dumb last night*. It is also advisable to comment on the person's behavior. Rather than saying *you're lousy* to your co-worker, you may instead say *your report was not well-written*. Always keep in mind that you must be considerate of other people's feelings.

Be firm.

The next step is being able to stick to your ideas, opinions, or wants. Many people may try to convince you to change your thoughts but you have to be firm by expressing your wants repeatedly. You may answer, *I still prefer to . . .* followed by a statement about your wants, ideas, or opinions. Others may make you feel guilty by accusing you of being inflexible or self-centered. Again, you deal with this by being firm. You may say *If conditions change tomorrow, then I might change my choice but at this time, this is what I want.* Never apologize for or be sorry about your views and preferences.

Anger Management

Anger management is simply expressing anger in a proper way at the right time and place. It doesn't mean that you should just keep your anger inside, allowing it to boil unexpressed. Unexpressed anger is harmful in itself because once the saturation point is reached, you might explode in an uncontrollable fashion. There are several ways of approaching and dealing with anger. You should 1) express your anger in private, 2) practice self-control, 3) cool down, 4) address the cause of anger after it is gone, 5) explore alternative behavior in showing or expressing anger.

Express your anger in private

Keep in mind that exploding in public is not appropriate. Showing your anger by lashing out at your children and spouse while in a grocery store or a public park is uncalled for, since you cannot achieve anything except hurt their feelings and harm your reputation. It is appropriate to express anger but it should be done for the right reason and in a proper way. If you cannot easily control your emotions, try expressing your anger in private by hitting a pillow, or a punching bag, shouting inside the bedroom or bathroom or writing your anger on a small piece of paper. You can also try communicating the reasons for your anger to a family member by talking about it and discussing it at home rather than flaunting it in public.

Practice self-control.

Try to avoid expressing your anger through humiliating or destructive behavior. Shouting at a person will further increase the communication gap and erode respect in the relationship. Hitting a person will not solve the problem but will more likely land you in jail. Control your impulses, and do not allow your emotions to control your thinking. Think first before you act in anger since the unwanted consequences might even include court appearances and possibly a prison sentence. Most importantly, any physical hurt and emotional pain caused by your display of anger will further unravel the thread that connects your relationship.

Cool down

Try your best to cool down before going any further in your discussion. Attempt to use a variety of techniques to release "steam," such as breathing exercises and progressive muscle relaxation. You can also attempt to stay away from the situation until you are less angry. You can do this by giving yourself a time-out, that is, going to a corner, a room, or any place where you can let your anger subside slowly. You can also try to divert your attention from the source of anger to a different form of physical or mental activity. For example, when you are angry, play basketball or try to complete your carpentry project.

Address the causes of anger

Address the causes of anger after the anger has gone. By this time, your mind is a lot clearer and perhaps more rational. Your emotions do not cloud your thinking anymore. This is the right time to figure out the sources of anger and possible solutions to it. If, for example, you get angry with a co-worker over work responsibilities, then talking to that person about it is appropriate. If open communication does not help, resolving the issue with your supervisor is the next move.

Explore alternative behavior

Expressing your anger appropriately includes asserting yourself rather than being aggressive, and diverting your energies from hurting someone to doing productive physical activity, such as exercising, cutting blocks of wood, and engaging in sports like basketball.

Improving Communication Skills

Many relationships have suffered miserably due to poor communication. I have seen couples in my clinic whose differences are minor but whose misunderstandings seem serious. They fight for the most trivial reasons and, most of the time, they do not know what they are fighting about. They have used a lot of energy to discredit each other but they fail to listen to each other, an act that requires significantly less energy. Techniques useful in improving communication are provided below.

Attempt to understand through active listening

The first step in improving communication is to attempt to understand through listening actively. As mentioned in the prior chapter, active listening requires frequent eye contact, use of appropriate gestures such as head nodding, and use of common, yet effective short statements such as *oh, ah, uh oh,* and so on. In these ways, you show that you are really listening. Acknowledging the other person's situation by repeating some of that person's statements also helps in establishing an alliance with the person.

Example:
> *I just can't get it. I can't understand why some people could be so mean. I thought she was my friend but now she spreads false rumors about me. I'm really mad.*

 That's certainly upsetting when you are talked about unfairly.

Free talk

Allowing the other person to talk not only improves understanding but also allows for a freer expression of feelings, ideas, and wants. People, when allowed to talk, feel that their thoughts and feelings are being valued and a feeling of importance, a vital ingredient of communication, is experienced.

Use empathic statements or gestures

The other person always appreciates acts of empathy. Although it's not always easy to show empathy (since many individuals are not "naturally" empathic), there are some techniques you can use. One technique is the use of empathic statements such as *it must have been upsetting for you, you've been through a lot, that's too bad, that's awful,* and *it's frustrating.* Another technique is the use of a pause or silence before making a response or comment. Please refer to Chapter 3 for details.

Avoid arguments and criticisms

Arguments, especially heated ones, are generally confrontational and insensitive. When you argue, you usually become bitter and fail to solve anything. Harsh criticisms likewise do not consider the emotions of other people and can result in hurt feelings. Polite or constructive criticism is more acceptable to the person being criticized. A better way of correcting behavior is by demonstrating the alternative or new behavior.

Example:
>Your ten-year-old son has the habit of banging the door late in the evening. Your other younger children are awakened by the loud noise. Instead of criticizing his behavior, you may show him politely how to close the door properly. Showing him the proper way each time he bangs the door can help to modify his behavior.

Express assertively your ideas/feelings/opinion/wants

Assertiveness is a necessary element of good communication. For detailed discussion, please see the assertiveness section above.

Time-Out

Time out is a technique that gives you a chance to escape from a complicated situation and confused thoughts, to reflect with a clear mind, and to control your emotions when pushed to their limits. Giving yourself time out requires: a) staying away from the situation, b) giving yourself time to reflect, c) escaping from routine, d) asking for help, and e) trying respite.

Stay away from the situation

When the situation gets tough emotionally and physically, it's about time to decide to get away. There is not much benefit "hanging in there" when things become uncontrollable and overwhelming. You need to keep your soul intact at a time when your emotional and physical health is on the brink of collapse. You don't have to wait for your health to deteriorate before you act. Decide now that this is the right time. Give yourself a chance to recover and reenergize.

Staying away does not always entail taking a long vacation or a visit to Arizona, although you may do so if you wish. Staying away can be an everyday matter. For example, suppose you and your wife are beginning to have a heated argument. Before everything gets out of hand, decide to stop the argument and isolate yourself in the bedroom for twenty minutes to cool off.

Give yourself time to reflect

One of the benefits of staying away from the situation is that it gives you time to think about and analyze your situation. You now have the opportunity to ask questions, and to consider fine points that are never allowed to surface at a time when you are too busy facing the grinds of daily living. You can now make queries such as: *how can I handle this situation better? Is it worth keeping the marriage intact? Or do I just have to move on? What have I done to start the fight? Do we need help?*

Escape from routine

Escaping from a stressful routine is a must. Escape need not be an expensive venture depleting your savings. Escape simply means making changes or diversions as the need arises. Such change can be done spontaneously everyday if need be. You may, for example, take walks during your break rather than go to the cafeteria. Or you may just stay in your office and do some breathing exercises or visualization. The frequency of escape will depend on your stress level, the amount of stressor, and how well you cope. In planning your escape, utilize some of the techniques discussed in this chapter and then determine what works. Just one hour of jogging or taking a different route each time is a big relief for some. One hour twice a day spent on your hobbies changes your perspective. Going to the spa even once a month provides comfort.

Ask for help

Sometimes, we need help from others when circumstances become overpowering. Do not hesitate to phone community agencies, support groups, mental health professionals, and churches.

Respite

Respite particularly applies to caregiving. You may need to coordinate with community agencies about providing your sick loved one with a daily home caretaker. Also, talk to your relatives about giving their time to help out on a daily or weekly basis. Consider utilizing personal home care on a temporary or permanent basis. When your sick family member requires more help than you and your relatives can provide, you may arrange for transfer to an appropriate care facility.

Scheduling Activities

Activity scheduling provides structure and focus. It keeps the person's mind preoccupied with some other activity. Scheduling activities helps to accomplish things, reinforces positive behavior, and contributes to the person's self-esteem. Moreover, establishing a routine and pursuing hobbies create diversion from the person's misery and change inactivity to productivity.

Example:
    Daily schedule
    8 A.M. Make the bed
    8:30 – 9:30 A.M. Prepare and eat breakfast
    9:30 – 11 A.M. Household chores (such as washing the dishes and cleaning the house)
    11 A.M. – 12:30 P.M. Prepare and eat lunch
    12:30 – 2 P.M. Afternoon nap
    2 – 3 P.M. Walking along the trail
    3 – 4 P.M. Rest and bath time
    4 – 6 P.M. Visit friends or family members
    6 – 7:30 P.M. Prepare and eat dinner
    7:30 – 9 P.M. Watch favorite TV show
    9 – 10 P.M. Reading Time
    10 P.M. Bedtime

Flexibility is important in creating a daily schedule. Modify your activities as you please. Allot more time for activities that give you a sense of well-being and provide personal meaning. Also, be realistic. Do not cramp a lot of activities in a span of a few hours since doing so may be detrimental to your physical health and may only stress you.

Time Management

There are two aspects to managing time. First, you list the things to do for the next few days, weeks, months or years, and then you prioritize the activities based on their importance and urgency. Include in the list those activities that give you the most personal satisfaction. For example, you have several to-do's on your list such as making the bed, getting the mail, paying bills, writing a chapter of your book, and studying for an exam. Then you schedule your day based on your priorities, such as deciding to write the chapter of the book first since there is a deadline to meet. Secondly, set your short-term and long-term goals and plan your activities around them. For example, you have three goals: first, to finish the book in three months; secondly, to lose weight about 10 lbs in a month; and thirdly, to read the entire Bible in one year. Your schedule will reflect these goals.

I have to emphasize the need to balance your priorities with family, recreational, and exercise programs. My personal conviction is that your family obligations should be at or near the top of the priority list. Including recreational and exercise programs in your routine is of course good for your mental and physical health.

Regular Physical Exercise

Regular physical exercise has been generally instrumental in establishing better mental health and self-esteem. A healthy body leads to a healthy mind, as the saying goes. There are several good reasons why regular physical exercise, such as jogging every morning, can help sick individuals. Exercise releases endorphin, a chemical released in your brain known to be more potent than some analgesics sold on the market. Endorphin gives the individual a sense of well-being. Aside from its endorphin-inducer function, exercise also releases tension from the muscles, relaxing the cells and sinews of your body. A daily exercise of only 25 minutes can go a long way in reducing stress and reinvigorating your system. As a result of its relaxing function, exercise can induce a more profound sleep and rest. Exercise, moreover, is a diversion from the grinds and demands of daily life. It encourages sick individuals to focus on improving their health, physically and mentally.

Recreational Activities

Recreational activities, such as hobbies, chores, and sports, offer advantages. First, they keep the mind occupied and stimulated. The mind is given the chance to explore, discover, look for answers, ask questions and simply enjoy the moment. Secondly, recreational activities help you focus on productive thoughts and endeavors. Instead of dwelling on thoughts about your traumatic or painful experiences, the mere act of being involved in the process – the movement, energy, effort, and struggle–gives you a respite from unproductive rumination. Thirdly, participating in various activities make productive use of your time. Doing a few things daily gives a sense of accomplishment. Just "lying around" does nothing to feed your self-esteem. Fourthly, being productive makes you feel good about yourself.

Sleep Hygiene

Sleep hygiene consists of steps to create a healthy sleeping habit. It involves things to do and to avoid – practical *do's and don'ts*. It does not include the use of sleeping medication as part of the exercise. You should:

- Avoid caffeinated foods, such as chocolates, and beverages such as soda, tea, and coffee, especially in the evening.
- Avoid afternoon naps, especially late afternoon naps such as after 3 or 4 pm.
- Use the bed only for sleeping and sex. Any other activity done in bed, such as watching TV and surfing the Internet, can only stimulate your senses and keep you awake. Reading, however, has induced a lot of people to sleep.
- Avoid recreational activities in the bedroom such as painting, drawing, and exercising.
- Avoid strenuous physical exercise, such as jogging, before going to bed since the activity releases a significant amount of adrenaline that stimulates your brain.
- Take stimulating medications, such as an antidepressant, in the morning rather than in the evening.
- Avoid stimulation at bedtime from any stimuli such as radio, television, and late visits by relatives.
- Do regular exercise and recreational activities during the day.
- Maintain your sleep schedule.

Living a Healthy Lifestyle

Nutritious food, regular exercise and recreational activities, sufficient sleep, ample worthwhile activities and avoidance of mood altering substances can provide a healthy way of living. Spirituality also provides tremendous comfort and hope. Just as your body and brain need nutritious food, your soul needs constant spiritual nourishment. Focus daily on ideas, literature, and activities that are uplifting and give meaning to your life.

Support Networks

Having relatives with you during difficult times is comforting. Support and reassurance from close friends and colleagues provide warmth and hope. It is crucial to establish support networks all the time regardless of your emotional state. Having someone to talk to is not only therapeutic but also preventative. They can give you advice during challenging times. Patients have told me how grateful they are to be surrounded by people who listen and care. Likewise, organizations and societies offer support groups, educational materials, respite, and other services to patients in emotional pain. Government agencies can also provide basic needs such as housing, financial assistance, food stamps, and the like. Together, family, friends, organizations, and government agencies can form a formidable team to prevent crisis and assist people face emergency.

Chapter 8

Depression

Case Scenario

Mr. S is a 45-year-old widower who just resigned as the CEO of a big private company. He was apparently doing well until about two months prior to consultation when he began to feel "down in the dumps" for no apparent reason. He stated that his work was stressful but manageable. Since he began to feel depressed, he became irritable when dealing with his co-workers. Subsequently, he noticed that he had to push himself to go to work in the morning. When at work for only a few hours, he easily got tired. Before this, he used to be very enthusiastic going to work and would work long hours. Now he felt different. He could not concentrate on his assigned task. At home, he just preferred to stay in bed with no interest to do anything, not even to cook his meals or wash the dishes.

Three weeks before his consultation, he began to isolate himself from everyone including close friends. Eventually, he stopped going to work. He frequently felt like crying. His sleep became worse. Interruptions and early awakening characterized his sleep. He could not eat properly since he lost his appetite. A week before consultation, the patient began thinking that he was better off dead. He felt worthless and helpless. He subsequently experienced severe guilt about his failed marriage, blaming himself for all that went wrong.

How is depression manifested?

Clinical depression is characterized by a combination of emotional, cognitive, physical and behavioral changes. Some patients have minimal symptoms, although others have serious ones. Feelings of sadness constitute the predominant symptom of clinical depression, and it is usually accompanied by one or more symptoms, as described below.

Emotional Changes

Sustained depression is frequently experienced as feeling "down in the dumps" or "feeling blue" for no apparent reason. It occurs frequently and at times may last the whole day. Patients complain about being tearful or wanting to cry. Others lose interest in routine activities including going to work, exercising, and performing basic chores. Depression is usually accompanied by irritability. Patients easily "snap" over trifles, reacting angrily to almost anything. As a consequence, conflicts with partners and co-workers are common occurrences. Moreover, patients tend to worry a lot, feeling on edge with "butterflies" in the stomach.

Behavioral changes

Significant impairment in functioning will occur if the depression is left untreated. Patients are unable to do basic tasks, including chores at home, and cannot perform satisfactorily at work. Difficulty with making the bed, doing the laundry, and even making phone calls becomes the norm. Agitation can occur and pacing back and forth at any time of the day is typical. A lack of desire for intimacy and sexual intercourse also accompanies depression. As a consequence, relational problems, especially between couples, ensue.

Physical and Cognitive Changes

Associated physical and cognitive symptoms occur. Sleep problems occur nightly so that going to sleep or maintaining sleep becomes a constant struggle. Some patients wake up early and cannot go back to sleep. Their energy becomes low and they complain of feeling weak and tired. It is common to hear, "I don't have any energy to do anything" from those suffering from depression. Likewise, concentration ability is problematic. Patients complain of an inability to focus at work. Watching television, reading books, and doing usual hobbies such as knitting or sewing, become laborious due to poor concentration. Memory lapses aggravate the patient's ability to think clearly. Forgetfulness is manifested in a variety of ways such as difficulty in remembering to take medication and problems with recalling names.

Appetite changes too. Some patients lose their appetite and consequently lose weight; others eat more when depressed and gain weight. Slowness in movement and thinking also occur, especially if the depression gets worse. Patients complain that moving the body becomes a struggle. Moreover, their thoughts don't come as smoothly and readily as before.

Psychological changes

Some patients feel worthless and have very poor self-esteem, feeling "rotten inside." Others feel guilty about something "terrible" they did in the past. Blame and rumination take place. Hopelessness is apparent when patients complain that there is "no light at the end of the tunnel." Moreover, they also feel that there is no one who can help them with their plight. Even the psychiatrists are not seen as a help. Such feeling of helplessness becomes pervasive as the illness gets worse. Thoughts of death eventually ensue if depression is allowed to worsen without any form of treatment. Some patients feel that life is not worth living anymore, that it makes more sense to die.

Case Scenario

Mr. S was advised to see a mental health professional by a friend but he decided to deal with it on his own. Several days later, he ended up staying longer in bed and he did not have enough energy even to take care of his personal hygiene. His tearfulness got worse. He lost a lot of weight. He gradually began thinking that he deserved to be sick because of the "sins" he had committed in the past. He became preoccupied with the notion that "hell" was his rightful place due to his misdeeds. One day, while lying down in bed, he heard a male voice telling him that he was better off dead. He initially disregarded the voice as "nonsense." Everyday his depression, suspiciousness and hearing "voices" became worse, however. Finally, the "voice" told him to cut his throat with a knife to attain "peace." He became so distressed that he phoned his sister about his experience. She decided to seek help for him.

What are the complications to anticipate?

Some seriously depressed patients develop unusual experiences such as delusions or inappropriate ideas or beliefs. Such ideas or beliefs are held with strong conviction, they do not conform to cultural norms, and they cannot be swayed by rational explanation. Such ideas include thoughts of deserving to die or having committed a grave sin in the past. Some patients harbor the thought that they have a terminal illness such as cancer or "rotting" intestines. Others are suspicious and think that people are talking about them behind their backs, or that people are laughing at them.

Auditory hallucination, although rare, has become distressful to many depressed patients. Hearing "voices," or "sounds" that others can't hear, can occur anytime during the day. These voices or sounds seem to come from the back of the head. Patients describe them as coming from either familiar or unfamiliar sources. Such "voices," coming from either male or female sources or at times, in combination, tell patients that they are "no good." Occasionally the voices command them to do certain things such as hurting themselves.

Patients' thoughts of death gradually turn worse and lead to suicidal thoughts and attempts. At first, the preoccupation occurs infrequently but later the thoughts of self-harm permeate the patient's daily life. Suicidal thoughts are present almost daily, at times the whole day consisting of a variety of plans on how to realize them effectively. Plans include overdosing on medications, cutting the wrist with a knife, hanging, or using a gun. Homicidal thoughts and attempts can occur in a severely depressed patient, and are occasionally associated with a false belief such as "saving the victim from the ills of the world."

Depression can also result in relationship problems because often the loved ones, including close friends, lack understanding about the illness and its impact on the patients functioning, behavior, and lifestyle. The illness causes disruption in familial, occupational, and social routine, and consequently conflict, loss of employment, separation and divorce may ensue. Furthermore, depression increases the risk of using illicit drugs and alcohol, perhaps in an attempt to self-medicate.

What are the common illnesses that show depression?

A variety of conditions can cause clinical depression. Medical conditions and medications are common culprits. In addition, major depressive disorder, bipolar disorder, dysthymic disorder, adjustment disorder, and premenstrual dysphoric disorder are known to involve depression.

Major Depressive Disorder

Major depressive disorder is a type of emotional illness that makes patients feel down, sad, or tearful on a regular basis. Such terrible feeling is associated with a) physical changes such as difficulty in sleeping, problems with concentration, lack of energy, and weight and appetite changes; and b) psychological changes such as feelings of hopelessness, helplessness, and worthlessness, or thoughts that life is not worth living anymore (DSM IV). Major depressive disorder may result in delusions, hallucinations, and suicidality or homicidality, especially at its worst phase. Depression associated with psychosis and substance/alcohol abuse increases the risk of suicide. This disorder occurs more frequently among women, with a 10-25% lifetime risk of developing the illness as opposed to a 5-12% risk for men. It can occur at any age, but the average onset is around 40 years old.

Regarding the cause of major depressive disorder, a strong genetic component is implicated as revealed by family and twin studies. A first-degree relative of a depressed patient has about twice the risk of developing the illness. Several biological factors are also implicated in its cause. Neurotransmitter or neurochemical abnormalities in the brain, especially involving serotonin, norepinephrine, dopamine, and acetylcholine, have been noted. In depressed patients with psychosis, brain imaging has shown inconclusive findings such as widening of the ventricles of the brain. Moreover, research reveals that stressors can precipitate major depression.

An untreated depression can last from six months to a year. Recurrence is also common. There is about a 30-50% chance of recurrence within two years of the illness. Treatment includes psychotherapy and antidepressants, such as venlafaxine, citalopram, and paroxetine. Occasionally hospitalization may be necessary.

DSM-IV Diagnostic Criteria for Major Depressive Episode

A. Five (or more) of the following symptoms have been present during the same 2-week period and represent a change from previous functioning; at least one of the symptoms is either 1) depressed mood or 2) loss of interest or pleasure. **Note:** Do not include symptoms that are clearly due to a general medical condition, or mood-incongruent delusions or hallucinations.

> 1) depressed mood most of the day, nearly every day, as indicated by either subjective report (e.g., feels sad or empty) or observation made by others (e.g., appears tearful) **Note:** In children and adolescents, can be irritable mood.
> 2) markedly diminished interest or pleasure in all, or almost all, activities most of the day, nearly every day
> 3) significant weight loss when not dieting or weight gain (e.g., a change of more than 5% of body weight in a month), or

decrease or increase in appetite nearly every day **Note:** In children, consider failure to make expected weight gains.
4) insomnia or hypersomnia nearly every day
5) psychomotor agitation or retardation nearly every day
6) fatigue or loss of energy nearly every day
7) feelings of worthlessness or excessive or inappropriate guilt (which may be delusional) nearly every day (not merely self-reproach or guilt about being sick)
8) diminished ability to think or concentrate, or indecisiveness, nearly every day
9) recurrent thoughts of death (not just fear of dying), recurrent suicidal ideation without specific plan, or a suicide attempt or a specific plan for committing suicide

B. The symptoms do not meet criteria for a Mixed Episode.
C. The symptoms cause clinically significant distress or impairment in social, occupational, or other important areas of functioning.
D. The symptoms are not due to the direct physiological effects of a substance or a general medical condition.
E. The symptoms are not better accounted for by Bereavement, i.e., after the loss of a loved one, the symptoms persist for longer than 2 months or are characterized by marked functional impairment, morbid preoccupation with worthlessness, suicidal ideation, psychotic symptoms, or psychomotor retardation.

Reprinted with permission from the Diagnostic and Statistical Manual of Mental Disorders, Fourth Edition, Text Revision. Copyright 2000 American Psychiatric Association.

Bipolar Disorder

Bipolar disorder is an illness consisting of episodes of depression and/or mania. Please see the description of the illness in the next chapter.

Dysthymic Disorder

Dysthymic disorder is mostly a chronic illness consisting of depression with low-level intensity. Such a feeling of depression is accompanied by physical changes, such as problems with sleep, concentration, appetite and energy, and psychological symptoms, such as a feeling of hopelessness. Patients with this disorder also complain of poor self-esteem (DSM IV). The illness has a 6% chance of developing in a lifetime and is common among women. Unmarried and young individuals are mostly affected.

The cause is not yet known but brain changes, such as the ones noted among patients with major depressive disorder and stressors, may be implicated. Because of its chronic course, significant problems in functioning, such as job loss and lack of interest in school, have been observed. Treatment includes antidepressants, such as fluoxetine or paroxetine, and psychotherapy.

Adjustment Disorder

Adjustment disorder is considered as the "development of emotional or behavioral symptoms in response to an identifiable stressor occurring within 3 months of the onset of the stressor" (DSM IV). Such changes include depression, tearfulness, excessive worrying, anger, agitation, and even behavioral problems such as aggression and drinking and driving. These symptoms, which may occur alone or in combination, can cause significant distress or functional impairment. Adjustment disorder is a common illness especially among adolescents. This illness may, however, happen to anyone exposed to familial, occupational, financial, interpersonal, academic, and other problems.

The prognosis is generally good since, for the most part, the emotional and behavioral difficulties may be resolved in three months after the onset of the stressor. Some patients, however, may develop a longer course and complications, such as depression. Treatment involves psychotherapy to help the patient deal with issues. Symptomatic treatment through the use of medication, such as temporary use of benzodiazepines for anxiety and agitation and occasional use of sleeping pill for insomnia may be considered.

Premenstrual Dysphoric Disorder

Premenstrual dysphoric disorder is an emotional illness associated with menstruation. Emotional and physical changes usually occur after ovulation up to the start of menstruation. The symptoms subside before the blood flow stops. The emotional change consists of depression, irritability, or anxiety. Physical changes include problems with appetite, sleep, concentration, energy, breast tenderness, and headache.

The etiology is not yet known. The course may be long-term. As for treatment, some patients benefit from selective serotonin reuptake inhibitors (SSRIs) such as fluoxetine.

Depression

Mood Disorder Due To General Medical Condition

Various medical conditions and their medications can cause depression. Brain tumor, stroke, epilepsy, hypothyroidism, systemic lupus erythematosus, and vitamin B-12 deficiency are some conditions that have been implicated. Medications that can cause depression include blood pressure medications such as propranolol and reserpine; steroids; antibiotics such as ampicillin; and analgesics such as Ibuprofen. Alcohol is also implicated.

Other Conditions Manifesting With Depression

A number of mental illnesses such as alcohol and substance abuse/dependence, generalized anxiety disorder, schizophrenia, phobia, personality disorders, dementia, and other major psychiatric disorders can also present with depression.

Early intervention

For Patient:

- Apply the HEAL technique.

- Accept depression, tearfulness, irritability, and other symptoms of depression. Consider them as manifestations of a medical illness that needs to be addressed.

- Deal with inappropriate thought via thought restructuring.
Example:
> Deal with rumination about your mistakes in past relationships by keeping yourself busy, such as making a quilt or focusing on the details of your latest project. Try to ignore the thought.

- For anxiety, use relaxation techniques such as breathing exercises and progressive muscle relaxation.

- Face anger and irritability through anger management.
Example:
> Before a potentially heated argument with your spouse starts, seclude yourself in the bedroom for several minutes until you cool down. Afterwards, you may decide to establish communication again to iron out some differences.

- For sleep impairment, practice sleep hygiene.

- For patients with low self-esteem, practice self-affirmation. Write in a notebook or journal at least three good things about yourself or at least three accomplishments daily. These positive comments need to be reviewed frequently. Also, dwell on positive experiences in the present and the past.

- Identify activities that make you feel better. If regular walks in the morning perk you up, then maintain this routine.

- Recognize and address the triggers of depression. Analyze your situation and the conditions that make you feel worse. By recognizing the cause, you may be able to take some preventive measures. If a conflict with your colleague precipitates your relapse, try to enhance your work relationship through improved communication.

- Cope with suicidal ideas through diversion: physical diversion involves activities such as recreational activities, outings, and exercise; social diversion includes visiting your friends and relatives; and mental diversion consists of mental activities such as thought replacement. Telling your relative and therapist about thoughts of self-harm is beneficial in getting immediate help.

- Ask for help and do not hesitate to call a hospital emergency room, crisis line, or mental health services.

- Ask for support from family members and relatives who are willing to share their resources if you can't solve your problem. For example, some may be willing to help you with a financial problem.

- Delay making major decisions while sick, such as divorce or selling the house. Usually a person can't make rational choices when the mind is impaired by the illness.

- Organize scheduled activities and routine.

- Avoid putting yourself down. Don't blame yourself for the miseries of others.

Depression

- Avoid the use of mood-altering substances such as alcohol and other illicit drugs as a way of dealing with the illness. Engaging in the use of substances can only add to the problem.

- Immerse yourself in pleasant and positive thoughts. Negative and self-critical thoughts will make you feel worse. Read positive literature that uplifts the spirit.

- Renew or strengthen your spirituality. Being connected with the higher power offers hope, inner confidence, guidance, and comfort.

For Caregivers:

- Apply the HELP method.

- Accept depression, tearfulness, irritability, and other symptoms of depression. Consider them as manifestations of a medical illness that needs to be addressed.

- Allow the person to talk and share emotions at a certain time of the day. At this time, focus on the patient's concerns and issues.

- Assist in getting support services and a mental health assessment by a professional. Offer to look for available mental health resources in the community and make the initial phone calls to set up an appointment.

- Help administer the medication prescribed by the physician (if the patient is unable to) or encourage medication self-management.

- Clarify safety by asking about the presence of suicidal or homicidal thoughts, intentions, or plans. Asking these questions will not push patients to hurt themselves or others.

- Be alert for signs of threat to self or self-destructive behavior such as superficial cuts on the wrist, empty bottles next to the bed, goodbye letters, giving away possessions, or taking a gun out of the cabinet. Be alert for any agitated or aggressive behavior as shown by pacing back and forth, easily getting upset for no reason, or becoming verbally abusive.

- Encourage the avoidance of mood-altering substances such as alcohol, and other illicit drugs as a way of coping with the problem. Remind the patient that using substances can only aggravate the situation.

- Call the hospital emergency room, crisis line, or the law enforcement agency for help if there is an imminent danger to the patient or others.

- Clarify treatment compliance. Ask the patient if he/she has been taking the medications prescribed by the physician.

- Ask for support from the family members. Help in conveying messages to friends and relatives. Some patients prefer to be in the company of caring people during these difficult times.

- Tell the patient to delay making major decisions while sick. Make the patient realize that sickness can impair one's judgment and hence can significantly impact on the patient's decision-making process.

- Reinforce coping skills and positive messages. Appreciate the patient's efforts in trying to help himself/herself such as through improved nutrition and sleep and participation in activities.

- Build the patient's hopes. Share your own experiences about how you successfully dealt with emotional difficulties in the past. Remind the patient that current difficulties are just temporary. If the patient has an appointment with a health care professional, reassure him/her that help is coming soon.

- Help patient organize activities and routine. Assist patients who lack the motivation and energy to establish structure by writing to-do lists and making appointments.

- Address low self-esteem: appreciate the patient's positive comments about oneself. Discourage or correct a low opinion of oneself. Avoid putting down the patient.

- Avoid arguments, confrontations, and criticisms. This is not the time to engage in fruitless communication.

- Help the patient in applying for sick or emergency leave.

Chapter **9**

Mania or Mood Swings

Case Scenario

Ms. S is a 29-year-old computer analyst who was her usual conservative and quiet self until about a month ago when she began to feel unusually happy. She felt three to five times stronger and believed that she was exceptionally beautiful. She did not know what triggered her recent emotion but admitted that her relationship with her childhood sweetheart had been on the rocks for the past year. Two weeks later, she claimed that she could influence the White House and change the US political landscape with just the wink of an eye. Her colleagues at work noticed that Ms S was very energetic, working from 5 AM until midnight without getting tired. Her work however was observed to be "sloppy" since she seemed to have difficulty attending to her tasks. She became talkative and most of the time she could not be interrupted. Her demeanor had changed. She started joking in a loud manner and frequently became sexually provocative.

Her concerned neighbor brought her to the nearest emergency room a few days ago after she drove 100 miles an hour in a quiet residential area. She almost hit an elderly woman who was crossing the street. On the same night, she hopped from one bar to another, and had sexual liaison with every "handsome man." She planned to get "serious" with one of them and to get married "before it's too late."

How is mania manifested?

Mania is characterized by a combination of emotional, cognitive, physical and behavioral changes. The predominant symptom is euphoria or the feeling of well-being. Some patients complain of irritability as the main problem. Mania is accompanied by one or more changes as described below.

Manic episode:

Emotional changes

As stated, a very common symptom is euphoria or a feeling of well-being. It is a feeling described as similar to being "high on drugs" since the patient feels "high" or unusually "happy" for no apparent reason. Unusual cheerfulness is also manifested when a patient laughs loudly, easily makes jokes about anything, and plays with words. Associated with the feeling of well-being is an increase in self-confidence. At this time, patients feel that they can do anything and that they have special abilities. Others show irritability and agitation rather than euphoria. These patients are hypersensitive, get upset quickly, and "snap" easily about trivial events.

Physical and Cognitive changes

Patients with mania experience a very high energy level, feel like "Superman," and believe they can work, play, or do other activities without needing rest or sleep. A few moments of rest replete their energy level without limit, making them excessively active almost all the time. Moreover, patients with mania show flight of ideas, that is, ideas that go from one topic to another without any logical or understandable connection between them. Others complain of racing thoughts. Distractibility or an inability to focus is common. Manic patients experience the urge to talk very rapidly and loudly, making them difficult to comprehend.

Behavioral changes

Patients who have the means spend "tons of money" at one time, sometimes spending their entire life savings. Buying sprees are not unusual. Involvement in new enterprises, business engagements, and dangerous activities, such as high-speed driving and one-night stands, are also common. Some patients can be hypersexual, that is, having sexual relations several times a day and occasionally with different partners.

Case scenario

Miss S was discharged from the emergency room after given a prescription for a mood stabilizer. After a few weeks of daily medication intake, she realized that the medication was making her "drowsy," and that it was not making her "happy." She decided to stop taking the pills so that she could regain the energy and happiness she had before the medication. Subsequently, she withdrew $30,000 from her savings to invest in a dotcom company. The next day she spent at least $5,000 for her business wardrobe. Having difficulty sleeping at night, she went to bars again, and drinking and sex became her routine. She stopped going to work since she assumed she didn't have to. When her co-worker phoned to inquire about her situation, she told her to "get lost," made threats and then slammed the phone down.

What are the complications to anticipate?

As a result of spending sprees and indiscriminate business transactions, patients have incurred financial burdens such as increasing debt and even bankruptcy. Unwanted pregnancies and sexually transmitted diseases may affect those who have sexual liaisons. Patients with tendencies to become agitated and violent have an increased risk of legal problems such as being charged with assault or uttering threats. Problems associated with speeding such as reckless driving and accidents are not uncommon. Suicidal ideas and attempts are sometimes found in those patients who become significantly depressed after the manic episode. Moreover, psychosis may occur.

What are the illnesses that manifest mania?

Primary psychiatric disorders, such as bipolar disorder and cyclothymic disorder, and certain kinds of medical conditions can manifest manic symptoms. The role of medical conditions and medication in causing manic-like symptoms should not be overlooked.

Bipolar Disorder

Bipolar disorder is another term for manic-depressive illness. During the depressed episode, the illness resembles the manifestation of major depression. The manic episode consists of various changes. For example, feelings of being exceptionally happy or irritable occur for several days. Such emotional change occurs along with physical changes such as sleep and concentration impairment, and behavioral changes such as talkativeness, restlessness, hypersexuality, and the pursuit of business and other entrepreneurial activities. Hypomanic episode may occur in lieu of mania but it is less intense (DSM IV). At its worse, some patients with bipolar disorder may experience delusions of grandeur which consist of inappropriate and unchanging ideas or beliefs. For example, they might think that they are *the messiah*, or the most trusted secret agents of the US President. Auditory hallucinations can also occur.

Both men and women have almost equal predilection. There is about a 0.4-1.0% risk of developing the illness in a lifetime. On the average, the onset occurs around 30 years old. A strong genetic component is involved in its cause. First-degree relatives of bipolar patients have about an18 times greater chance of developing the disorder. Brain studies have shown inconclusive results such as widening of ventricles (CT Scan Head) and increase of lesions in the white matter area (MRI). The role of stressors is also implicated in precipitating the illness.

Bipolar disorder is a recurring illness that mostly starts with a depressed phase followed later by an episode of mania, most likely within two years. The average number of episodes in a patient is about nine. When untreated, the illness can last as long as three months. Treatment includes mood stabilizers, such as lithium and valproic acid and psychotherapy. Some patients require hospitalization.

DSM-IV Diagnostic Criteria for Manic Episode

A. A distinct period of abnormally and persistently elevated, expansive, irritable mood, lasting at least 1 week (or any duration if hospitalization is necessary).

B. During the period of mood disturbance, three (or more) of the following symptoms have persisted (four if the mood is only irritable) and have been present to a significant degree:

    1) inflated self-esteem or grandiosity

    2) decreased need for sleep (e.g., feels rested after only 3 hours of sleep)

    3) more talkative than usual or pressure to keep talking

    4) flight of ideas or subjective experience that thoughts are racing

    5) distractibility (i.e., attention too easily drawn to unimportant or irrelevant external stimuli)

6) increase in goal-directed activity (either socially, at work or school, or sexually) or psychomotor agitation
7) excessive involvement in pleasurable activities that have a high potential for painful consequences (e.g., engaging in unrestrained buying sprees, sexual indiscretions, or foolish business investments)

C. The symptoms do not meet criteria for a Mixed Episode.

D. The mood disturbance is sufficiently severe to cause marked impairment in occupational functioning or in usual social activities or relationships with others, or to necessitate hospitalization to prevent harm to self or others, or there are psychotic features.

E. The symptoms are not due to the direct physiological effects of a substance or a general medical condition. **Note:** Manic-like episodes that are clearly caused by somatic antidepressant treatment (e.g., medication, electroconvulsive therapy, light therapy) should not count toward a diagnosis of Bipolar I Disorder.

Reprinted with permission from the Diagnostic and Statistical Manual of Mental Disorders, Fourth Edition, Text Revision. Copyright 2000 American Psychiatric Association.

Cyclothymic Disorder

Cyclothymic disorder is considered a mild type of bipolar disorder since it consists of hypomanic (less intense mania) and low-level depressive symptoms. These symptoms are thus lower in intensity than those of bipolar and major depressive disorders. About 3-10% of all patients seen in the outpatient clinic may suffer from this type of disorder.

Biological factors are implicated as a cause. About 30% of patients suffering from this disorder have family members with bipolar disorder. The disorder usually starts early in life, when patients are in their teens. Friends and relatives occasionally describe these individuals as "moody." Treatment consists of mood stabilizers, such as lithium and valproic acid, and psychotherapy.

Schizoaffective Disorder

Schizoaffective disorder is a type of psychotic disorder that presents with manic symptoms. (Please see its description in Chapter 15).

Mood Disorder due to Substance or General Medical Condition

Medical and neurologic conditions, such as stroke, brain trauma, kidney failure, hyperthyroidism, and vitamin B-12 deficiency, can cause manic symptoms. Medications and illicit drugs are also implicated, including captopril, methylphenidate, cocaine (illegal drug), opiates, and cimetidine.

Early intervention

For patients:

- Apply the HEAL technique.

- Accept irritability, excessive energy, hypersexuality, delusions of grandeur, and other symptoms of manic/depression as part of the illness.

- For anxiety, use relaxation techniques such as breathing exercises and progressive muscle relaxation.

- Face anger and irritability using anger management.
Example:
> You are told that you're becoming "snappy." You also realize that you get angry over the smallest things. Try to control yourself before saying anything against a person. Closely listen to the words coming from your mouth. Stay away from a situation that easily irritates you.

- For sleep impairment, do sleep hygiene.

- Recognize and address the triggers of mania. By recognizing the cause, you may be able to take some preventive measures. If a conflict with your colleague precipitates your relapse, try to improve your work relationship through better communication.

- Closely observe yourself. Be alert for signs of threats to yourself or self-destructive behavior such as excessive spending, promiscuity, poor business decisions, goodbye letters, giving away possessions, taking a gun out from the cabinet, and speeding. Be alert for any agitated or aggressive behavior such as by pacing back and forth, easily getting upset for no reason, and becoming verbally abusive and violent.

- Cope with suicidal thoughts through physical, mental, and social diversions. Inform a close friend or relative and discuss thoughts of self-harm.

- Address your impulsive behavior by first analyzing its risk and benefits. Think before acting.

- Comply with the medication and treatment prescribed by your physician.

- Avoid using mood-altering substances such as alcohol and other illicit drugs because these substances will only complicate your illness and your life.

- Check for the presence or worsening of symptoms. For example, you are becoming more impulsive and physically assaultive.

- Ask for support from the family. Some relatives are willing to share their resources and their time.

- Establish a routine of activities to which you can direct your excess energy. Activities include playing ball, jogging, and walking.

- Express your emotions to trusted friends and relatives.

- Delay making major decisions, such as establishing businesses, divorcing your spouse, and resigning from a job. You can make better decisions when you get well.

- Apply for sick or emergency leave.

- Deal with inappropriate thoughts through thought restructuring.

- Immerse yourself in pleasant and positive thoughts. Negative and self-critical thoughts will obviously make you feel worse.

- Renew or strengthen your spirituality. Being connected with the higher power offers hope, inner confidence, guidance, and comfort.

For Caregivers:

• Apply the HELP method.

• Accept irritability, excessive energy, hypersexuality, delusions of grandeur, and other symptoms of manic/depression as part of the illness.

• Help administer the medication prescribed by the physician, if the patient is unable to.

• Be alert for signs of threats to self or self-destructive behavior such as superficial cuts on the wrist, empty bottles, excessive spending, promiscuity, deleterious business decisions, goodbye letters, giving away possessions, taking a gun out of the cabinet, and speeding. Be alert for any agitated or aggressive behavior such as pacing back and forth, easily getting upset for no reason, becoming verbally abusive, and physically assaultive.

• Clarify safety by asking about the presence of suicidal or homicidal thoughts. Asking this question will not push patients to hurt themselves or others.

• Encourage the avoidance of mood-altering substances such as alcohol and other illicit drugs. Remind the patient that using substances can only aggravate the situation.

• Check for the presence or worsening of symptoms. For example, the patient is increasingly becoming psychotic with delusions of grandeur and becoming physically assaultive.

• Call for help from a hospital emergency room, crisis line, and law enforcement officers if there is an imminent danger to self or others or an inability to take care of self.

• Clarify treatment compliance. Make sure that the patient takes the medication regularly.

• Contain inappropriate behavior such as being disruptive in public places, speeding, and sexual promiscuity, if at all possible. You may do this by keeping car keys, encouraging the patient to stay at home, and taking the patient to a hospital.

- Ask for support from family members. Assist the patient in conveying messages to friends and relatives. Some patients prefer to be in the company of caring people during these difficult times.

- Encourage the patient to establish a routine and a schedule of activities.

- Allow the patient to express emotions at a certain time of the day and focus on his/her concerns and issues. Try to set limits since these patients tend to talk too much. Be cordial and polite in terminating a conversation.

- Monitor spending and other impulsive behavior and assist patient in weighing the advantages and disadvantages of the behavior.

- Tell the patient to delay making major decisions while sick such as establishing businesses, traveling with no definite destination, and divorcing a spouse.

- Help the patient to apply for sick or emergency leave.

- Avoid arguments, confrontations, and criticisms. These actions are self-defeating.

- Reinforce coping skills and positive messages. Appreciate patients' efforts in trying to help themselves such as through improved nutrition and sleep, participation in recreational activities.

- Help the patient organize scheduled activities and routine. Assist patients, who lack the motivation, to establish structure by writing to-do lists and making appointments.

Chapter 10

Panic Attacks

Case Scenario

Mr. Y, a 26-year-old truck driver, was doing well until six weeks ago when he suddenly experienced an "overwhelming" sensation while driving his truck. He stopped the vehicle. His heart pounding and his chest tight, he feared that he was having a heart attack. He could hardly breathe. The "overwhelming" experience ended after about twenty minutes but he was already sweating profusely. While on his way, Mr. Y decided to visit an emergency room for a check up. His blood tests, electrocardiogram, and other tests showed normal results. He left the hospital reassured. However, the next few days were not easy for him. He feared that he would experience the same "attack" again. He had been preoccupied with it for several days until one night, while watching television at home, he again felt the sudden rush of chest pounding and tightness. He was sweating and trembling, and had difficulty in breathing. He thought he was going to die.

How is panic attack manifested?

Panic attack:

Emotional and Cognitive changes

Panic attacks involve various symptoms. Patients frequently experience an overwhelming and rapid rush of severe distress. At this time, they are terrified that something very bad is going to happen. Typically, they fear that a heart attack, stroke, mental breakdown, or even death is imminent. There seems to be no clear trigger or precipitant for such uncomfortable feelings. The symptoms, however, go as fast as they come. Typically, the discomfort, fear, and associated physical changes (as noted below) last for approximately thirty minutes, although some patients experience the symptoms longer.

Physical changes

During the attack, patients experience trembling or shaking sensation from head to toe. Sweating occurs in the whole body, and the arms and feet experience "pins and needles sensations." Heart pounding and palpitations accompany chest heaviness and patients also experience a breathing difficulty which makes them distraught and uncomfortable. At times, a feeling of choking prevents patients from eating. Due to these symptoms, patients usually end up in the hospital emergency room with the thought that "something physical" is going on. During evaluation by health care professionals, fast heartbeats are noted but otherwise patients generally show no medical problems.

Case scenario

Mr. X became "fearful" of going outside his house. He felt safer having the "attack" at home. Initially, he made excuses to avoid going back to work. Later, he decided that he wasn't fit to be working and he quit. He had several attacks at home as well as while standing in line at the grocery store. Thereafter Mr. X felt desperate about his situation. He visited his family physician who prescribed a medication, but after a trial of a few weeks, he felt the medication was "useless." He stopped taking the medication and decided to deal with the attacks on his own. He began to drink alcohol heavily, which temporarily relieved some of his fear.

What are the complications to anticipate?

Patients who develop panic attacks outside the house (in the mall, in the car, or inside the elevator) begin to fear going to these places. Patients dread or stop traveling, confining themselves in their homes. Going to work or even buying necessities become almost impossible. Given a choice, patients avoid places where the likelihood of obtaining help or escaping is perceived as difficult, such as being in a crowd and driving in a tunnel. Agoraphobia often occurs.

To help themselves overcome their problems, some patients choose self-medication. They take alcohol or use street drugs just to attain the usual "normal" feeling that make them functional and that has eluded them since the onset of the attack. Eventually, they use these substances excessively, to the point where they develop a new problem: substance abuse and dependence. Patients with panic attacks have an increased risk to develop clinical depression, resulting in further impairment. This combination of panic and depression is unfortunate since the potential for suicidal ideation and gesture is heightened.

What are the illnesses that show panic attacks?

Panic disorder, phobia, alcohol and illicit drug use, and a variety of mental and medical conditions can involve panic attacks.

Panic Disorder

Panic disorder is an emotional illness characterized by the presence of a **panic attack,** which is described as "a discrete period of intense fear or discomfort in which . . . symptoms develop abruptly and reach a peak within 10 minutes" (DSM IV). Such distress or discomfort is associated with several physical changes such as chest discomfort, sweating, tremulousness, dizziness, and palpitations. The first attack is usually not precipitated by any stimuli and occurs spontaneously. Symptoms generally last for about thirty minutes. Panic attacks are recurrent. Patients generally develop agoraphobia, a condition in which the patient experiences feelings of helplessness, distress, and discomfort being in certain situations such as tunnels, bridges, and elevators. They also perceive that escape from these situations might be difficult so they try to avoid them. If they cannot, they need to be with someone who accompanies and reassures them. The lifetime chance to develop panic disorder stands at 1.5-5%, while for agoraphobia, it is 0.6-6%. On average, the onset occurs around age 25.

In terms of etiology, several studies have shown that panic disorder has a strong genetic component. First-degree relatives of panic disorder patients have about 4-8 times the risk of developing the illness. Brain imaging has demonstrated a temporal lobe dysfunction especially in the hippocampus area. Moreover, neurotransmitter (serotonin, norepinephrine, and GABA) dysregulation is also implicated.

Panic disorder is generally a chronic illness since, on long-term follow-up, about 50% of panic patients still have minimal symptoms. However, about 30-40% completely recover.

DSM-IV Diagnostic Criteria for Panic Attack

A discrete period of intense fear or discomfort, in which four (or more) of the following symptoms developed abruptly and reached a peak within 10 minutes:
1) palpitations, pounding heart, or accelerated heart rate
2) sweating
3) trembling or shaking
4) sensations of shortness of breath or smothering
5) feeling of choking
6) chest pain or discomfort
7) nausea or abdominal distress
8) feeling dizzy, unsteady, lightheaded, or faint
9) derealization (feelings of unreality) or depersonalization (being detached from oneself)
10) fear of losing control or going crazy
11) fear of dying
12) paresthesias (numbness or tingling sensations)
13) chills or hot flushes

DSM-IV Diagnostic Criteria for Panic Disorder Without Agoraphobia

A. Both 1) or 2)
1) recurrent unexpected Panic Attacks
2) at least one of the attacks has been followed by 1 month (or more) of one (or more) of the following:
    a) persistent concern about having additional attacks
    b) worry about the implications of the attack or its consequences (e.g., losing control, having a heart attack, "going crazy")
    c) a significant change in behavior related to the attacks
B. Absence of Agoraphobia.
C. The Panic Attacks are not due to the direct physiological effects of a substance or a general medical condition.

D. The Panic Attacks are not better accounted for by another mental disorder, such as Social Phobia (e.g., occurring on exposure to feared social situations), Specific Phobia (e.g., on exposure to a specific phobic situation), Obsessive-Compulsive Disorder (e.g., on exposure to dirt in someone with an obsession about contamination), Posttraumatic Stress Disorder (e.g., in response to stimuli associated with a severe stressor), or Separation Anxiety Disorder (e.g. in response to being away from home or close relatives).

Both criteria are reprinted with permission from the Diagnostic and Statistical Manual of Mental Disorders, Fourth Edition, Text Revision. Copyright 2000 American Psychiatric Association.

Phobia

Both specific and social phobia can cause panic attacks. Phobic patients may develop the panic attack when they are exposed to the stimuli that cause intense fear and anxiety. (More detailed information can be found in Chapter 11.)

Panic Attacks due to Medical Condition or Medications

Several medical conditions such as ischemic heart disease, hypoglycemia, pulmonary embolism, and hyperthyroidism can cause panic attacks. Moreover, medications, such as amphetamine and caffeine, or withdrawal from drugs such as benzodiazepine or alcohol, may cause the attack.

Other conditions

Panic attacks may also appear in patients with major depressive disorder, posttraumatic stress disorder, adjustment disorder, and bipolar disorder.

Early intervention:

For Patients:

- Apply the HEAL technique.

- Accept the signs and symptoms of panic attacks and deal with them.

Panic Attacks

- Deal with inappropriate thoughts through thought restructuring. If, for instance, you remain preoccupied with the thought of having another attack, apply thought replacement and mental diversion accordingly. Focus your attention and energies on worthwhile undertaking.

- Apply breathing exercises and other relaxation techniques to prevent impending attack or to reduce the intensity of an ongoing attack.

- Confront the fear of and preoccupation with panic attacks through diversion.
Example:
> Each time you begin to be preoccupied with having a panic attack, divert your attention to a hobby or physical exercise, and keep yourself busy by doing chores at home.

- Identify other effective coping strategies such as the so-what technique, progressive muscle relaxation, and visualization of pleasant scenery.
Example:
> Each time you feel that you are going to have a panic attack, tell yourself "So what, I know it's not going to kill me."

- Establish and organize daily schedule of activities that include exercise, hobbies, and socialization. Identify activities that make you feel better. If carpentry or gardening helps you, establish this routine.

- Comply with the medication and treatment recommended by the physician.

- Cope with suicidal ideas through physical, mental, and social diversions. Tell a close friend and relative and talk about thoughts of self-harm.

- Closely observe yourself. Be alert for signs of threats to yourself or self-destructive behavior, such as writing goodbye letters, giving your possessions away, taking a gun out of the cabinet, and taking unprescribed pills.

- Avoid the use of mood-altering substances such as alcohol and other illicit drugs as a way of dealing with the illness. The use of substances only adds to the problem.

- Call a hospital emergency room, crisis line, or mental health services for help.

- Delay making major decisions while sick, such as resigning from your job, cutting ties with relatives, or engaging in unproductive activities.

- Ask for support from family members who can provide comfort and reassurance.

- Practice sleep hygiene for sleep problems.

- Talk about concerns with trusted friends and relatives.

- Apply for sick or emergency leave, if necessary.

- Renew or strengthen your spirituality. Being connected with the higher power offers hope, inner confidence, guidance, and comfort.

For Caregivers:
- Apply the HELP method.

- Accept the signs and symptoms of panic attacks.

- Assist the patient in learning and mastering coping strategies, such as breathing exercises, progressive muscle relaxation, systematic desensitization, and visualization.

- Clarify treatment compliance. Help administer the medication prescribed by the physician. Encourage the patient to take the medication and to visit the physician or therapist.

- Encourage the avoidance of mood-altering substances such as alcohol and other illicit drugs as a way of coping with problems. Remind the patient that using substances only aggravates the situation.

- Clarify safety by asking about the presence of suicidal or homicidal thoughts. Asking this question will not push patients to hurt themselves or others.

- Check for the presence or worsening of symptoms such as serious panic attacks, severe impairment in functioning, and inability to leave the house.

- Ask for support from family members. Some patients prefer to be in the company of caring people during these difficult times.

- Allow the patient to talk about concerns and emotions at a certain time of the day.

- Encourage the patient to see a health care professional immediately if that patient has not received professional help for a worsening illness.

- Avoid arguments, confrontations, and criticisms. This is not the best time to engage in fruitless communication.

- Advice the patient to delay making major decisions while sick such as resigning from the job, cutting ties with relatives, or engaging in unproductive activities.

- Build up the patient's hopes. Share your own experiences or the experiences of others. Remind the patient that current difficulties are just temporary. If the patient has an appointment with a health care professional, then you reassure him/her that help is coming soon.

- Appreciate patients' positive comments about themselves. Discourage any low opinions they have of themselves. Avoid criticizing a patient.

- Help the patient to apply for sick or emergency leave. Offer to fill out forms or write letters.

- Help the patient organize a routine or schedule of activities. Assist patients who lack the motivation to establish structure by writing to-do lists and making appointments.

Chapter 11

Phobia

Case Scenario

Mrs. X is a 42-year-old scientist who decided to see a mental health counselor after advice from her laboratory supervisor. She reported that since her teen-age years she had been suffering from a fear of rats. She related that this fear started after she and her family visited an old cabin in the country when she was nineteen. While cleaning the bedroom, she saw a large rat jumping off the drawer. She was terrified and screamed uncontrollably for several minutes before calming down. Her family members thought that she overreacted to the event. But for Mrs. X, the image of the rat lingered until they left for the city.

Despite having an occasional fear of seeing another rat, she moved on with her life. She finished college in four years and has worked as a scientist ever since. Several months ago however, she was assigned to conduct drug research in a laboratory using rats as subjects. She thought that she had gotten over her fear of rats until one day, while at the laboratory, she could hardly approach the experimental rats to do her observation and the administration of the drug. She was fearful and felt very agitated. She left the laboratory without doing her tasks. Subsequently, the symptoms persisted and the research was delayed. Her supervisor then asked her to seek help.

How is phobia manifested?

Phobia has an emotional component related to exposure to stimuli or events such as the one mentioned above. The emotional component includes excessive fear, anxiety, or distress. Such emotional problems happen during exposure or anticipating exposure to certain situations or events such as high places, being in a crowd, speaking or eating in front of an audience, and riding in a plane. Particular animals, such as a dog, cat, and rat can cause a phobic reaction, as well as other circumstances such as exposure to blood. Patients are considerably relieved once the dreaded stimuli are taken away. Moreover, avoidance of the feared event or situation is a natural consequence.

Case scenario

Mrs. X went back to work after only a few sessions with the therapist. She thought that the therapy sessions were simply a "waste of time." After a brief review of her new research assignment with the supervisor, she headed to the rat laboratory right away. As soon as she opened the door, she felt nauseated by the smell of the rats. Inside, she began to feel an "overwhelming sense of fear." She wanted to scream but she couldn't. She was "paralyzed" just looking at the rats and couldn't perform her tasks that day. Frustrated about her situation, she went home. The next few days were worse. She felt "out of it" and was unable to do her assignment, despite some help from her supervisor. The symptoms persisted causing further delays, and her employer decided to let her go. She was advised to look for a research job with no exposure to rats.

What are the complications to anticipate?

Impairment in performance at work or in any situation may occur. Patients suffer particularly if their phobia is connected to their occupation, such as in the example above. Those individuals who are required to speak in public, yet suffer from fear of speaking before an audience, are likewise significantly affected. Eventually, if the illness remains untreated, patients' personal and social functioning suffer.

What are the illnesses that show phobia?

The common kinds of phobia include social phobia, specific phobia, and agoraphobia.

Social phobia

Social phobia is a type of illness in which a social situation, such as speaking in public or eating in front of strangers, is dreaded and if possible avoided. The exposure to the situation causes severe anxiety, discomfort or distress. Patients with this disorder harbor the thought that their behavior or mannerisms in a social context is embarrassing. Some fear that they will make mistakes and be disgraced. About one third of the patients develop major depression. The lifetime chance to develop social phobia is from 3 to 13%.

The disorder is more common among women than men. On average, the illness starts during teenage years. A strong genetic component is implicated in its cause. First-degree relatives of phobic patients have three times the risk of developing the illness. Treatment includes medication such as selective serotonin reuptake inhibitors (SSRI) and behavior therapy.

DSM-IV Diagnostic Criteria for Social Phobia

A. A marked and persistent fear of one or more social or performance situations in which the person is exposed to unfamiliar people or to possible scrutiny by others. The individual fears that he or she will act in a way (or show anxiety symptoms) that will be humiliating or embarrassing. **Note:** In children, there must be evidence of the capacity for age-appropriate social relationships with familiar people and the anxiety must occur in peer settings, not just in interactions with adults.
B. Exposure to the feared social situation almost invariably provokes anxiety, which may take the form of a situationally bound or situationally predisposed Panic Attack. **Note:** In children, the anxiety may be expressed by crying, tantrums, freezing, or shrinking from social situations with unfamiliar people.
C. The person recognizes that the fear is excessive or unreasonable. **Note:** In children, this feature may be absent.
D. The feared social or performance situations are avoided or else are endured with intense anxiety or distress.

E. The avoidance, anxious anticipation, or distress in feared social or performance situation(s) interferes significantly with the person's normal routine, occupational (academic) functioning, or social activities or relationships, or there is marked distress about having the phobia.

F. In individuals under age 18 years, the duration is at least 6 months.

G. The fear or avoidance is not due to the direct physiological effects of a substance or a general medical condition and is not better accounted for by another mental disorder.

H. If a general medical condition or another mental disorder is present, the fear in Criterion A is unrelated to it, e.g., the fear is not of Stuttering, trembling in Parkinson's disease, or exhibiting abnormal eating behavior in Anorexia Nervosa or Bulimia Nervosa.

Reprinted with permission from the Diagnostic and Statistical Manual of Mental Disorders, Fourth Edition, Text Revision. Copyright 2000 American Psychiatric Association.

Specific Phobia

Specific phobia denotes irrational fear associated with an exposure to certain stimuli such as insects, water, elevators, driving, and blood. Such exposure creates unwarranted distress, anxiety, and discomfort. Avoidance of the feared situation significantly affects the individual's functioning. According to Kaplan and Sadock, specific phobia is the most common mental disorder among women, and second most common among men. The illness has about an 11% risk of developing in a lifetime. The illness may develop between the age of 5 and 9 but some patients acquire the illness in their twenties. This disorder is known to run in the family. Behavior therapy is the treatment of choice.

Agoraphobia

This topic is discussed in Chapter 10.

Early intervention

For Patients:
- Apply the HEAL technique.

- Accept the signs and symptoms of phobia and deal with them.

- Deal with inappropriate thoughts through thought restructuring.
Example:
> You have a fear of flying and the thought of traveling brings substantial distress and anxiety. Get information on the incidence of air accidents. You learn that the chance of plane crash is very low. You then reassure yourself through repetitive self-talk that flying is safe.

- Practice exposure and desensitization regularly.
Example:
> <u>Fear of Flying</u>
>
> First, virtually expose yourself to the plane by visualizing yourself arriving in the airport, walking to the security area, being in the waiting area, walking towards the plane, then being inside the plane, and finally by enjoying the scenery while looking through the plane window. Repeat the exercise several times until mastery. Once you have mastered this virtual exposure, proceed with the next phase. Secondly, actually expose yourself to the airport, by watching planes come and go, then by going inside the airport several times, followed by sitting for a while in the waiting area. You may do this exercise before the scheduled flight.
>
> Frequent flying will certainly help you. You can also first put yourself in a relaxed state through relaxation techniques before the virtual and actual exposures.

- Identify effective coping methods and deal with anxiety through relaxation strategies such as the visualization of peaceful scenery, progressive muscle relaxation, and breathing exercises.

- Confront fear with diversion.
Example:
> When fear of flying starts to set in, try talking various topics with your companion or the person sitting beside you. By doing this, you shift your focus from yourself to the other person.

- Comply with the medication and treatment recommended by your physician.

- Avoid the use of mood-altering substances such as alcohol and other illicit drugs as a way of dealing with the illness because their use only adds to the problem.

- Check for presence or worsening of symptoms, such as extreme fear and anxiety which result in significant impairment in functioning.

- Call hospital emergency room, crisis line, and mental health services for help.

- Establish a daily routine and schedule that include exercise, hobbies, and socialization.

- Ask for support from the family. Some relatives are willing to share their time and resources.

- Talk about concerns with trusted friends and relatives.

- Avoid putting yourself down.

- Delay making major decisions, such as resigning from a job, while sick.

- Apply for sick or emergency leave, if necessary.

- Recognize the advantages and disadvantages of the phobic behavior.

- Renew or strengthen your spirituality. Being connected with the higher power offers hope, inner confidence, guidance, and comfort.

For Caregivers:

- Apply the HELP method.

- Accept the signs and symptoms of phobia and help patient deal with them.

- Help and reinforce the patient in learning and mastering coping strategies such as breathing exercises, progressive muscle relaxation, systematic desensitization, and visualization.

- Help administer the medication prescribed by the physician.

- Encourage the avoidance of mood-altering substances such as alcohol and other illicit drugs as a way of coping with the problem. Remind the patient that using substances can only aggravate the situation.

- Check for the presence or worsening of symptoms such as an inability to go outside the house and any significant impairment in functioning.

- Clarify treatment compliance. Ask the patient if a regular visit with a health care professional has been followed.

- Ask for support from the family members. Some patients prefer to be in the company of caring people during these difficult times.

- Allow the patient to talk about concerns and issues.

- Appreciate patients' efforts to help themselves such as through improved nutrition and sleep, and participation in recreational activities.

- Encourage the patient to see a physician or mental health professional.

- Avoid arguments, confrontations, and criticisms. This is not the best time to engage in fruitless communication.

- Address the patient's low self-esteem and appreciate the patient's positive comments about self. Correct low opinion of self if possible. Avoid putting down the patient.

- Tell the patient to delay making major decisions while sick such as resigning from a job.

- Build the patient's hopes. Share your own experiences or the experiences of others in dealing successfully with the illness. Remind the patient that current difficulties are just temporary. If the patient has an appointment with a health care professional, then assure him/her that help is coming.

- Help the patient in applying for sick or emergency leave.

- Assist in getting support services and a mental health assessment by a professional.

- Help the patient organize activities and routine. Assist patients who lack the motivation to establish structure by writing to-do lists and making appointments.

Chapter 12

Obsessions and compulsions

Case Scenario

Mr. Y, a 24-year-old college student, was abused sexually as a child. He was doing well until about two years ago when he developed a compelling need to wash his hands repetitively. He reported that initially he was washing his hands about ten to twenty times a day. However, the hand washing gradually became more pronounced and reached a point where he would spend most of his time in front of the faucet. His repetitive hand washing resulted in superficial wounds on his hands. Despite his efforts to wash and their consequences, he still felt that his hands were dirty. Thus he had no choice but to wash his hands again and again for several hours.

A few months later, he had to wash not just his hands but also the faucet for fear that it was also contaminated. He used antibacterial spray repeatedly to "clean the dirty faucet." He thought that if he stopped cleaning, he would die of bacterial infection. He also had an intrusive thought that "something terrible" would happen to his girlfriend if he stopped washing. Despite his efforts to counter these thoughts with "something positive," he couldn't really get rid of them. A month before seeing a psychiatrist, Mr. Y decided to wash not only his hands but also his entire body. He would spend at least 5 hours per day in the shower.

How is the illness manifested?

This type of illness has two components: obsession and compulsion.

Obsessions

Obsessions are repetitive thoughts considered to be excessively annoying, disturbing, and bothersome. These "unnecessary" thoughts cause a significant level of emotional distress, such as anxiety, especially when they keep coming back despite the patient's attempt to suppress their appearance. Examples include homosexual, blasphemous, and murderous thoughts. One female college student had thoughts of performing oral sex on a saint. A religious mother of two had unwanted thoughts of having sex with her female colleague. Other inappropriate and repetitive thoughts include thoughts of being dirty and of having excessive doubt. Some patients experience a repetitive appearance of unwanted and disgusting images. A single 24-year-old mother, for example, had images of pushing her two-year-old son from their fourth floor apartment. A male personnel manager had images of stabbing himself with a Swiss knife. Thoughts of using profane words toward loved ones can also be found. For example, a male patient wanted to say "fuck you" or "shit" each time he saw his mother.

Almost all patients wrestle with these thoughts through various techniques such as by replacing the "nasty thoughts, words, or images" with pleasant and acceptable ones. Some try hard to prevent their appearance by blocking them from their consciousness. But the majority of patients have difficulty countering them, some getting worse in the effort. As a result, patients experience guilt and depressed feelings. Moreover, patients exhibit "obsessive slowness" particularly if they become meticulous and repetitive about the details of an otherwise routine activity.

Compulsions

Compulsions are recurrent actions and "mental acts" performed to relieve emotional distress resulting from the inappropriate thoughts. Hand washing, for instance, is performed to reduce the anxiety related to the thought of being "dirty." In addition, repetitive checking occurs to reassure the person experiencing severe doubt. As the level of distress increases, the more patients are compelled to perform the behavior. In general, compulsive behavior is what the person is forced to do in order to feel better and to achieve a short-term respite from the bothersome thoughts.

Case scenario

Mr. Y remained symptomatic despite being on SSRIs. However, he developed intolerable side effects and decided to stop taking these medications. Two months later, he went back to his routine of washing his hands repetitively and taking a shower for longer periods. He couldn't attend his classes anymore since he was spending most of his time in the bathroom. His body developed superficial wounds due to the excessive use of soap and the frequent rubbing with a hand towel. Many times during his bathing periods, he would run out of hot water and would use cold water to wash his body. One day, he was rushed to the emergency room with low body temperature.

What are the complications to anticipate?

Obsessions and compulsions are debilitating especially if allowed to progress without any intervention by mental health professionals. The severe forms of this mental problem may cause significant impairment in patients' functioning. A substantial number of patients cannot do their usual activities since their waking hours are consumed by the repetitive reenactment of thoughts and behavior. One patient, for instance, spent one third of her waking hours in the bathroom, taking a bath for fear of dying from the "dirt." One male patient cleaned his house with Chlorox the whole day. Patients are unable to start or finish a project when they become meticulous and preoccupied with details of a project or an activity.

Physical problems may result from the patients' rituals. Wounds and excoriations can occur after excessive washing. Occasionally, hypothermia or low body temperature can result from taking a long bath.

What illnesses manifest with obsession and compulsion?

Several psychiatric and medical conditions have shown obsession and compulsion. Obsessive and compulsive disorder (OCD) is the primary psychiatric illness that manifests this type of illness. OCD can also co-exist with other psychiatric disorders such as major depressive disorder and schizophrenia. Medical problems have likewise been implicated in the appearance of these symptoms.

Obsessive-Compulsive Disorder

Obsessive-compulsive disorder is a type of illness manifested by either obsession, or compulsion, or both. Obsession consists of repetitive "thoughts, impulses, or images that are experienced . . . as intrusive and inappropriate and that cause marked anxiety or distress." The patients with obsession make an effort to stop or even counteract the repetitive and unwanted experience. Compulsion, on the other hand, refers to recurring actions, behavior, or even "mental acts" that patients are compelled to perform in order to prevent or reduce anxiety or distress (DSM IV). Patients identify the symptoms as "absurd." Contamination and doubt are the two most common obsessions, with washing and checking as the most common compulsions respectively.

This disorder has a 2-3% chance of developing in a lifetime. In adults, both men and women have equal predilection. The illness may develop at about the age of twenty. OCD has a strong genetic component as a cause. Biological factors, such as serotonin, reduction of the size of the caudate as shown by brain imaging, and increase in metabolism and blood flow in some areas of the brain (revealed by PET Scan), have a role in its etiology.

Stress can precipitate or aggravate the OCD symptoms. Usually the course is chronic, especially since there is a delay of several years before patients seek help. OCD patients have the potential to develop depression or be involved in suicidal behavior. However, about 20-30% of patients significantly improve with treatment involving medication, such as SSRIs, and behavior therapy.

DSM-IV Diagnostic Criteria for Obsessive-Compulsive Disorder

A. Either obsessions or compulsions:
Obsessions as defined by 1), 2), 3), and 4):
      1) recurrent and persistent thoughts, impulses, or images that are experienced, at some time during the disturbance, as intrusive and inappropriate and that cause marked anxiety or distress
      2) the thoughts, impulses, or images are not simply excessive worries about real life problems
      3) the person attempts to ignore or suppress such as thoughts, impulses, or images, or to neutralize them with some other thought or action
      4) the person recognizes that the obsessional thoughts, impulses, or images are a product of his or her own mind
Compulsions as defined by 1) and 2):
      1) repetitive behaviors (e.g., hand washing, ordering, checking) or mental acts (e.g., praying, counting, repeating words silently) that the person feels driven to perform in

response to an obsession, or according to rules that must be applied rigidly

2) the behaviors or mental acts are aimed at preventing or reducing distress or preventing some dreaded event or situation; however, these behaviors or mental acts either are not connected in a realistic way with what they are designed to neutralize or prevent or are clearly excessive

B. At some point during the course of the disorder, the person has recognized that the obsessions or compulsions are excessive or unreasonable. **Note:** This does not apply to children.

C. The obsessions or compulsions cause marked distress, are time consuming (take more than 1 hour a day), or significantly interfere with the person's normal routine, occupational (or academic) functioning, or usual social activities or relationships.

D. If another Axis I disorder is present, the content of the obsessions or compulsions is not restricted to it.

E. The disturbance is not due to the direct physiological effects of a substance or a general medical condition.

Reprinted with permission from the Diagnostic and Statistical Manual of Mental Disorders, Fourth Edition, Text Revision. Copyright 2000 American Psychiatric Association.

Other Mental Disorders Manifesting Obsession or Compulsion

Obsessive-compulsive disorder occurs in the presence of other psychiatric disorders such as schizophrenia, major depressive disorder, social phobia, and panic disorder. Patients with an eating disorder appear to be obsessed with their weight and how they look (See chapter 17 for details). Impulse control disorders, such as kleptomania, trichotillomania, pathologic gambling, and paraphilia appear to manifest some form of obsession or compulsion. These illnesses are associated with the experience of pleasure. A patient with paraphilia, for instance telephone scatologia, considers having sex on the phone as pleasant and pleasurable rather than as a distressful and anxiety-provoking event. Likewise, a patient who is "obsessed" with gambling enjoys the thrill, the "chase," and the wins associated with the activity. However, marked anxiety, anger, and at times depression become a consequence of losing a lot of money since debts and family conflict ensue.

Obsessions and Compulsions

Medical Conditions that Present With Obsession Or Compulsion

Tourette's Disorder and complex partial seizure can manifest with obsession and compulsion. Tourette's Disorder manifests with tics, a long-term disorder presenting with repetitive and sudden stereotyped movements (e.g. frequent eye blinking or grimacing) and vocalization (e.g. sniffing or barking). A complex partial seizure is a neurologic disorder associated with a range of changes, from simple movements such as chewing or lip smacking, to more complex behavior which may involve driving, disrobing, or walking.

Early Intervention

For Patients:

- Apply the HEAL technique.

- Accept the signs and symptoms of obsession and compulsion and deal with them.

- Deal with inappropriate thoughts through thought restructuring.
Example:
> Each time the intrusive thoughts occur (such as murderous thoughts), suddenly change your focus to an object or event you see in front of you, or quickly replace it with a different thought.

- Practice exposure and response prevention regularly. Response prevention is simply a behavioral intervention that requires you not to give in to the urge of performing rituals, actions, or behavior in reaction to the obsession. You are stopping yourself from following your urges and rituals.
Example:
> Each time you develop the urge to perform a ritual or action, such as checking the doorknob in reaction to the obsession (doubt), decide instead to do a chore, for instance vacuuming the floor. Focus intently on what you are doing.

- Establish a routine and daily schedule that includes exercise, hobbies, and socialization.

- Identify effective coping and relaxation strategies such as diversion, visualization of peaceful scenery, progressive muscle relaxation, and breathing exercises.

• Comply with the medication and treatment recommended by your physician.

• Avoid the use of mood-altering substances such as alcohol, and other illicit drugs as a way of dealing with the illness. They only add to the problem.

• Check for the presence or worsening of symptoms, such as prolonged (several hours) and more frequent hand washing or checking which indicate significant impairment in functioning.

• Call a hospital emergency room, crisis line, or mental health services for help.

• Ask for support from family. Some relatives are willing to share their time and resources.

• Talk about your concerns with trusted friends and relatives.

• Avoid putting yourself down.

• Delay making major decisions, such as resigning from a job, while sick.

• Recognize the advantages and disadvantages of the behavior. Once you recognize that the disadvantages outweigh the advantages, decide to stop.

• Renew or strengthen your spirituality. Being connected with the higher power offers hope, inner confidence, guidance, and comfort.

For Caregivers:
• Apply the HELP method.

• Accept the signs and symptoms of obsession and compulsion and assist the patient in dealing with them.

• Help and reinforce the patient in learning and mastering coping strategies such as breathing exercises, progressive muscle relaxation, exposure and response prevention.

• Help administer the medication prescribed by the physician.

Obsessions and Compulsions

- Encourage the avoidance of mood-altering substances such as alcohol, and other illicit drugs as a way of coping with the problem. Remind the patient that using substances only aggravates the situation.

- Check for the presence or worsening of symptoms, such as serious preoccupation with the intrusive thoughts and significant impairment in functioning.

- Clarify treatment compliance.

- Ask for support from family members. Some patients prefer to be in the company of caring people during these difficult times.

- Allow the patient to talk about concerns and issues.

- Encourage the patient to see a physician or mental health professional.

- Avoid arguments, confrontations, and criticisms. This is not the best time to engage in fruitless communication.

- Tell the patient to delay making major decisions such as resigning from a job, while sick.

- Build the patient's hopes. Share your own experiences or relate the experiences of others who have successfully dealt with the illness. Remind the patient that current difficulties are just temporary. If the patient has an appointment, reassure him/her that help is coming.

- Appreciate the patient's positive comments about self. Correct patient's low opinion of himself/herself. Avoid putting the patient down.

- Help the patient apply for sick or emergency leave.

- Help the patient organize daily activities and routines. Assist patients who lack the motivation to establish structure by writing to-do lists and making appointments.

Chapter 13

Emotional Difficulties After a Trauma

Case Scenario

Ms. T, a 26-year-old social worker, has worked with sexually abused children for the past six months. She was her usual self until about four months ago when she began to experience nightmares of being molested. She felt that her nightmares were triggered by the incessant stories of abuse in the workplace. In her childhood, her uncle who lived in the basement of their home raped her. She remembered waking up with the full weight of her uncle on top of her. She wanted to scream but he threatened to slash her throat with a knife. He had forced her to do certain "things" for many years until she finally told her parents about it. Her uncle was subsequently evicted from the house. Ms. T received therapy for almost a year and she thought that she was fine.

Since she started working with abused children, she had felt uncomfortable. Occasionally, she would cry after listening to their horrifying experiences. A few months ago, she experienced nightmares almost daily about her being raped and fearing for her life. Moreover, she experienced flashbacks about the incident with her uncle. Each time she walked by a place that reminded her of the rape, she would feel uncomfortable and fearful.

Subsequently, she felt "dirty and sick" each time she and her boyfriend had sex. Her job was also affected since she couldn't focus anymore.

How is the illness manifested?

This illness presents with two vital components. First, there is the occurrence of trauma. Secondly, the traumatized individual develops emotional, behavioral, and physical changes as a result of the trauma.

Trauma

The trauma that occurs is considered life threatening, causing extreme fear in the individual and frequently resulting in physical injury. Examples of trauma include rape, frequent sexual or physical abuse, and exposure to severe violence and death, such as being in the battlefield.

Changes after the trauma

The changes in the traumatized individual can occur after several days, months or even years after the trauma. The prominent symptom is the recurrence or the reliving of the trauma in the form of nightmares, dreams, and frequent recollections of the event. The nightmares and dreams may not necessarily mimic the specific event, but the individual may experience the same theme of a life-threatening event, with the fear and distress involved in the original trauma. Eventually, patients develop emotional problems such as fear, anxiety, depression, and irritability, especially when reminded of the trauma. Complaints of sadness and excessive worry occur. Physical changes include concentration difficulty which prevent patients from focusing on their tasks and interrupted sleep.

Traumatized individuals develop behavioral changes such as excessive alertness or hypervigilance. For example, a woman who was recently raped frequently looks out her windows and checks the door locks when at home, or she looks behind her back when walking. Cognitive changes such as an inability to remember portions of the trauma, and thoughts of deserving it or being responsible for it, are also common. Moreover, patients avoid reminders of the trauma – an activity, person, situation, place, smell, and so on. For example, a young woman who was raped in a dark area of a mall avoids shopping. Lovemaking with her boyfriend also causes distress and fear since the act reminds her of the incident. Any reminders of the trauma, such as the scent of a perfume and the smell of a person's hair, are dreaded.

Case scenario

Ms. T eventually became depressed about her situation. She began to experience sleep problems. Her interest in going to work was low and she had to push herself just to get up in the morning. Her appetite suffered significantly and she lost about 30 lbs. For the past few weeks, her relationship with her boyfriend had turned from bad to worse since he had difficulty dealing with her irritability and inability to function sexually. They finally broke up after she caught him having an affair with her best friend. Subsequently, she became more depressed and had more nightmares. She preferred to stay in bed and contemplated ending her life. Her brother came to visit one day and saw her in that depressed state. She was eventually brought to the hospital for further treatment.

What are the complications to anticipate?

Patients' relationships suffer because of the various changes that occur in the individual after the trauma. Mood changes such as irritability can cause friction and can trigger unnecessary arguments. If clinical depression occurs along with the other symptoms, the whole picture becomes more complicated. Suicidal thoughts and gestures resulting from severe depression and feelings of worthlessness may ensue. Trouble with the law may occur, especially among patients who self-medicate on alcohol or on other mood-altering substances. Drunk driving and violent or agitated behavior are not uncommon.

What are the illnesses manifesting with emotional difficulties after a trauma?

There are two major psychiatric disorders associated with trauma: posttraumatic stress disorder and acute stress disorder.

Posttraumatic Stress Disorder

Posttraumatic stress disorder (PTSD) is an illness manifested by emotional difficulties related to a traumatic experience. The trauma (mostly overwhelming experience, such as rape for women, and war for men), which is considered a precipitant of this illness, may have occurred a few weeks or a number of years before the onset of emotional changes. The condition encompasses emotional changes (anger, depression, anxiety, paranoia, panic attacks, hypervigilance, and fear) and various recall behavior (nightmares, dreams, recollection, and flashbacks) about the event or any related event. In addition, patients with PTSD experience changes in their sleep and eating patterns and an inability to focus on tasks at hand. This disorder has a 1-3% chance of developing in a lifetime and appears to be common among individuals living alone such as widows or divorcees, and among those with a low income.

Several factors are implicated in its etiology. Genetic predisposition, prior trauma, current stressors, and relationship problems predispose certain individuals to this type of psychiatric disorder. Some neurotransmitter changes, such as those of norepinephrine and dopamine, have been observed. About 30% of PTSD patients eventually recover. Those patients with strong support from their families and with good personality traits prior to the illness have a good prognosis. Treatment includes SSRIs and psychotherapy.

DSM-IV Diagnostic Criteria for Posttraumatic Stress Disorder

A. The person has been exposed to a traumatic event in which both of the following were present:
> 1) the person experienced, witnessed, or was confronted with an event or events that involved actual or threatened death or serious injury, or a threat to the physical integrity of self or others.
>
> 2) the person's response involved intense fear, helplessness, or horror. **Note:** In children, this may be expressed instead by disorganized or agitated behavior

B. The traumatic event is persistently reexperienced in one (or more) of the following ways:
> 1) recurrent and intrusive distressing recollections of the event, including images, thoughts, or perceptions. **Note:** In young children, repetitive play may occur in which themes or aspects of the trauma are expressed.
>
> 2) recurrent distressing dreams of the event. **Note:** In children, there may be frightening dreams without recognizable content.
>
> 3) acting or feeling as if the traumatic event were recurring. **Note:** In young children, trauma-specific reenactment may occur.
>
> 4) intense psychological distress at exposure to internal or external cues that symbolize or resemble an aspect of the traumatic event.
>
> 5) physiological reactivity on exposure to internal or external cues that symbolize or resemble an aspect of the traumatic event.

C. Persistent avoidance of stimuli associated with the trauma and numbing of general responsiveness (not present before the trauma), as indicated by three (or more) of the following:

    1) efforts to avoid thoughts, feelings, or conversations associated with the trauma
    2) efforts to avoid activities, places, or people that arouse recollections of the trauma
    3) inability to recall an important aspect of the trauma
    4) markedly diminished interest or participation in significant activities
    5) feeling of detachment or estrangement from others
    6) restricted range of affect (e.g., unable to have loving feelings)
    7) sense of a foreshortened future

D. Persistent symptoms of increased arousal (not present before the trauma), as indicated by two (or more) of the following:

    1) difficulty falling or staying asleep
    2) irritability or outbursts of anger
    3) difficulty concentrating
    4) hypervigilance
    5) exaggerated startle response

E. Duration of the disturbance (symptoms in Criteria B, C, and D) is more than 1 month.

F. The disturbance causes clinically significant distress or impairment in social, occupational, or other important areas of functioning.

Reprinted with permission from the Diagnostic and Statistical Manual of Mental Disorders, Fourth Edition, Text revision. Copyright 2000 American Psychiatric Association.

Acute Stress Disorder

Acute stress disorder is related to PTSD, and both have the same manifestations and cause. The difference between the two disorders lies in the time frame. While PTSD occurs after one month, acute stress disorder (ASD) occurs within a month of the trauma and its duration does not exceed four weeks after the trauma.

Early intervention

Emotional Difficulties After a Trauma

For Patients:
- Apply the HEAL technique.

- Accept irritability, tearfulness, nightmares, flashbacks, depression, and other symptoms associated with the trauma and deal with them.

- Address the issues immediately, such as reporting the incident to appropriate authorities.

- Review any helpful coping strategies in the past that can be applied at present. If talking to close friends was previously helpful, then you may still use this coping strategy.

- Recognize changes in emotion and behavior including the presence of nightmares or re-experiencing the traumatic event in everyday life.

- Think of ways to protect yourself and reassure yourself about safety. For example, install an alarm or put double locks on your doors.

- Have plenty of rest, nutritious food, and sleep.

- Check for any change in emotion or behavior when exposed to a situation similar to the traumatic event. Avoid places that cause severe distress during the initial stage of the illness or difficulty.

- Comply with the medication. Make sure that you take the medication regularly as prescribed by your physician.

- Deal with anger and irritability through anger management.
Example:
> Release your anger by punching the pillow or shouting in your bedroom. Having a good cry also helps.

- For sleep problems, apply sleep hygiene.

- Deal with anxiety through the use of relaxation techniques such as breathing exercises, visual imagery, and progressive muscle relaxation.

- Deal with inappropriate thought via thought restructuring.
Example:

If you begin to blame yourself for the incident, engage in self-talk that does not put the blame on you, such as "I tried to fight him off but that guy was stronger than me."

• For patients with low self-esteem, practice self-affirmation. Write in a notebook or journal at least three good things about yourself daily. These positive comments need to be reviewed frequently. Also, dwell on positive experiences in the present and the past. Read positive literature that uplifts the spirit.

• Identify activities such as exercise, socialization, diversion, and recreational activities that make you feel better. If regular walks in the morning perks you up, then establish this routine.

• Recognize and address the triggers of depression. By recognizing the cause, you may be able to create preventive measures. If a conflict with your colleague, for instance, precipitates your relapse, try to improve your work relationship through improved communication.

• Cope with suicidal ideas through diversion: physical diversion involves activities such as recreational activities, going out, and exercise; social diversion includes visiting your friends and relatives; and mental diversion consists of mental activities such as thought replacement. Telling your relatives and therapist about thoughts of self-harm is beneficial in getting immediate help.

• Call a hospital emergency room, crisis line, or mental health services for help.

• Ask for support from family members. Some relatives are willing to share their resources and time. They may be willing to accompany you and give you comfort.

• Delay making major decisions while sick, such as resigning from a job. The majority of people can't make rational choices when their minds are impaired by the illness.

• Organize daily activities and routine.

• Avoid putting yourself down and don't blame yourself for what happened.

Emotional Difficulties After a Trauma

- Avoid the use of mood-altering substances such as alcohol and other illicit drugs as a way of dealing with the illness. Their use only adds to the problem.

- Attempt to immerse yourself in pleasant and positive thoughts. Negative and self-critical thoughts will make you feel worse.

- Address fear-provoking situations through gradual exposure. Example:
    > If sexual assault occurred in a basement, the thought of going to the basement would elicit fear and anxiety. Such emotional difficulties intensify when you are actually exposed to the place of trauma. Address this issue by gradually exposing yourself to the place.

- Renew or strengthen your spirituality. Being connected with the higher power offers hope, inner confidence, guidance, and comfort.

For Caregivers:

- Apply the HELP method

- Accept tearfulness, irritability, nightmares, flashbacks and other symptoms related to trauma. Consider them as manifestations of an illness that must be addressed.

- Assist the patient in getting a mental health assessment by a professional, in being involved in support groups, and accessing services, including an emergency room or a visit to a physician for a medical/psychiatric assessment.

- Help the patient organize personal undertakings such as paying bills, making an appointment with a lawyer, and so on.

- Allow the patient to talk about the details of the traumatic event.

- Provide comfort and help so that the patient feels safe and secure.

- Help the patient report an incident, e.g., rape, to appropriate authorities.

- Advise the patient not to put blame on self.

- Encourage plenty of rest, nutritious food, and sleep.

- Allow the person to talk and share emotions at a certain time of the day and focus on the patient's concerns and issues.

- Help administer the medication prescribed by the physician (if patient is unable to) or encourage medication self-management.

- Be alert for signs of threat to self or self-destructive behavior such as superficial cuts in the wrist, empty bottles next to the bed, goodbye letters, giving away possessions, taking a gun out of the cabinet. Be alert for any agitated or aggressive behavior as shown by pacing back and forth, getting upset for no reason, and becoming verbally abusive.

- Clarify safety by asking about the presence of suicidal or homicidal thoughts. Asking this question will not push patients to hurt themselves or others.

- Encourage the avoidance of mood-altering substances such as alcohol and other illicit drugs as a way of coping with the problem. Remind the patient that using substances only aggravates the situation.

- Clarify treatment compliance. Ask the patient if he/she has been taking the medications prescribed by the physician.

- Ask for support from family members. Help in conveying messages to friends and relatives. Some patients prefer to be in the company of caring people during these difficult times.

- Tell the patient to delay making major decisions while sick. Make the patient realize that sickness can impair one's judgment and hence can adversely affect the decision-making process.

- Reinforce coping skills and positive messages. Appreciate patients' efforts to help themselves such as through improved nutrition and sleep, and participation in recreational activities.

- Build the patient's hopes. Share your own experiences about how you successfully dealt with emotional difficulties in the past. Remind the patient that current difficulties are just temporary. If the patient has an appointment, stress that help is coming soon.

- Offer to look for available mental health resources in the community and make the initial phone calls to set up an appointment

- Help the patient organize a schedule of activities and routine. Assist patients who lack the motivation and energy to establish structure by writing to-do lists and making appointments.

- Address low self-esteem and appreciate patients' positive comments about themselves. Correct patients' low opinion of themselves. Avoid putting patients down.

- Avoid arguments, confrontations, and criticisms. This is not the best time to engage in fruitless communication.

- Help the patient in applying for sick or emergency leave.

Chapter 14

Anxiety

Case Scenario

Mr. Z, a 46-year-old businessman, was his usual self until about nine months prior to consultation when he began to worry about "trifles." He used to be a "happy-go-lucky" guy who took everything in stride. But nine months ago, he felt "butterflies" in his stomach almost every day and lasting the whole day. He worried about everything – clothes to wear, his daughter's birthday party, his son's coming home late, his performance at work, and other "small things." His colleagues at work noticed his inability to focus on details. Prior to these worry problems, he was known as an "expert" for details. A few months ago, he began to experience agitation and restlessness. He felt tense almost all the time. Despite feeling tired the whole day, he could hardly sleep at night. His wife observed that he would repetitively pace in the bedroom and worry excessively.

Mr. Z remembered that his mother had the same "nerve problems" in the past and never got any treatment. Instead, she drank a lot of alcohol to calm her nerves. Her drinking had affected him emotionally. As a child, he developed episodes of anxiety especially when going to school.

How is the illness manifested?

Anxiety disorder is manifested by predominantly emotional and physical changes. The predominant symptom consists of extreme worrying or anxiety, along with one or more symptoms described below.

Emotional Changes

Patients develop significant or overwhelming worry or anxiety about almost anything. Patients tend to be preoccupied with finances even if money is not a problem, with employment even if work has not produced any stress, about their health and that of their closest relatives, and about the safety of their children and grandchildren. Closest relatives and spouses describe patients as "worry warts," worrying excessively for no reason. They have difficulty relaxing, as if always on edge and tense. Pacing back and forth while preoccupied is common.

Physical Changes

Some patients exhibit a significant decrease in concentration ability. Since they are too concerned with their worry, they cannot concentrate on tasks at hand, whether at work or at home. Sleep problems also occur. Patients report difficulty falling asleep and tossing and turning most of the night. Others have interrupted sleep, waking up in the middle of the night. Still other patients wake up early in the morning and cannot go back to sleep. When patients cannot go to sleep, they end up worrying more.

Other physical changes may include sweating and having tremors of the hands and lips if their anxiety is sufficiently intense.

Case scenario

Mr. Z felt he could handle the problem on his own. He bought and tried to read several self-help books on anxiety and relaxation techniques. Despite his efforts, his anxiety episodes became worse. He was almost "paralyzed" because he could not do anything for fear that his performance would result in something "really awful." He gradually stopped going to work. During evaluation in the psychiatrist's clinic, he was sweating, agitated, and complained of a severe upset stomach. He couldn't stay still.

What are the complications to anticipate?

Patients who worry a lot develop significant impairment in functioning. Some patients cannot go to work anymore because they worry about having an accident or car trouble on the way, about having an argument with a co-worker, about doing a poor job on an assigned task, or about coming to work late. At home, patients' functioning is also substantially limited by the illness. Because of excessive preoccupation with worry, patients cannot complete basic tasks at home, such as cleaning the house, making the bed, doing the laundry, or preparing meals.

What illnesses manifest with chronic anxiety?

Primary psychiatric illness (such as generalized anxiety disorder) and medical disorders (for instance thyroid dysfunction and hypoglycemia) have resulted in chronic anxiety.

Generalized Anxiety Disorder

Generalized anxiety disorder or GAD is a type of long-term illness manifested by unnecessary and extreme worrying about "trifles" or small things that others do not usually worry about. Such feelings of anxiety are associated with physiologic changes such as sweating and palpitations, and other physical symptoms such as agitation or restlessness, sleep and concentration problems, and occasionally sensations of shortness of breath. GAD has about a 45% chance of developing in a lifetime. The majority of patients suffering from GAD also suffer from other mental disorders such as major depressive disorder and panic disorder. GAD is more common among women than men. Stressors may precede its onset. The illness can develop in childhood.

GAD has a strong genetic component as shown by twin studies. Biological factors, such as neurotransmitter (serotonin, norepinephrine, and others) dysregulation in some areas of the brain, including the basal ganglia and frontal cortex, and decrease in metabolism in the basal ganglia as shown by a PET scan, have also been implicated as a possible cause. Treatment includes psychotropic medication such as buspirone, SSRIs, benzodiazepines, and psychotherapy.

DSM-IV Diagnostic Criteria for Generalized Anxiety Disorder

A. Excessive anxiety and worry (apprehensive expectation), occurring more days than not for at least 6 months, about a number of events or activities (such as work or school performance).
B. The person finds it difficult to control the worry.
C. The anxiety and worry are associated with three (or more) of the following six symptoms (with at least some symptoms present for more

days than not for the past 6 months). **Note:** Only one item is required in children.
      1) restlessness or feeling keyed up or on edge
      2) being easily fatigued
      3) difficulty concentrating or mind going blank
      4) irritability
      5) muscle tension
      6) tension disturbance
D. The focus of the anxiety and worry is not confined to features of an Axis I disorder.
E. The anxiety, worry, or physical symptoms cause clinically significant distress or impairment in social, occupational, or other important areas of functioning.
F. The disturbance is not due to the direct physiological effects of a substance or a general medical condition and does not occur exclusively during a Mood Disorder, a Psychotic Disorder, or a Pervasive Developmental Disorder.

Reprinted with permission from the Diagnostic and Statistical Manual of Mental Disorders, Fourth Edition, Text Revision. Copyright 2000 American Psychiatric Association.

Anxiety Disorder Due to General Medical Condition

Medical illnesses can present with anxiety symptoms. Thyroid and parathyroid dysfunction, cardiac arrhythmias, Sjogren's syndrome, hypoglycemia, and other conditions cause anxiety symptoms. Alcohol and illicit drugs such as cocaine and LSD also induce substantial worry.

Other Psychiatric Conditions

GAD can usually co-exist with other major mental disorders such as major depressive disorder, panic disorder, and alcohol dependence.

Adjustment Disorder

Any stressors such as a conflict with spouse, legal trouble, and financial problems may cause excessive anxiety resulting in functional dysfunction and distress. As mentioned earlier, the symptoms should resolve within three months after the stressor ceases. (See the discussion on adjustment disorder in Chapter 8.)

Early intervention

For Patients:

• Apply the HEAL technique.

• Accept signs and symptoms of anxiety and deal with them.

• Recognize and address the triggers of anxiety. Apply problem-solving strategies if appropriate.
Example:
> You realize that since you developed financial difficulties, you have become a worry wart. You then decide to look for ways to solve the problem. You look at various alternatives such as looking for a job and asking for temporary government assistance. After weighing the pros and cons, you choose to look for a job in the city.

• Deal with inappropriate thoughts through thought restructuring.
Example:
> You have become a chronic worrier. As a result, your functioning and physical health has been greatly affected. You decide to closely weigh the advantages and disadvantages of worry in your life. After analysis, you realize that worry has not helped you in any way. You decide to stop worrying and begin to say "enough is enough."

• Establish a routine and schedule activities that include exercise, hobbies, and socialization. Identify any activities that make you feel better.

• Identify effective coping and relaxation strategies such as visualization of peaceful scenery, progressive muscle relaxation, and breathing exercises.

• Comply with the medication and treatment recommended by your physician.

- Avoid the use of mood-altering substances such as alcohol and other illicit drugs as a way of dealing with the illness. The use of these substances only adds to the problem.

- Check for the presence or worsening of symptoms, such as severe restlessness, inability to concentrate and sleep, and others resulting in significant impairment in functioning.

- Call a hospital emergency room, crisis line, or mental health services for help.

- Ask for support from family members who are willing to share their time and resources.

- Talk about concerns with trusted friends and relatives.

- Avoid putting yourself down.

- Delay making major decisions, such as resigning from a job, while sick. Many people can't make rational choices when their mind is impaired by the illness.

- Apply for sick or emergency leave, if necessary.

- Recognize the advantages and disadvantages of the behavior. If the disadvantages outweigh the advantages, decide to stop the behavior.

- For sleep problems, apply sleep hygiene.

- Renew or strengthen your spirituality. Being connected with the higher power offers hope, inner confidence, guidance, and comfort.

For Caregivers:

- Apply the HELP method.

- Accept the signs and symptoms of anxiety. Consider them as manifestations of an illness that must be addressed.

- Assist in getting support services and a mental health assessment by a health care professional. Offer to look for available mental health resources in the community and make the initial phone calls to set up an appointment.

• Help and reinforce the patient in learning and mastering coping strategies such as breathing exercises, progressive muscle relaxation, systematic desensitization, and visualization.

• Help administer the medication prescribed by the physician.

• Encourage the avoidance of mood-altering substances such as alcohol and other illicit drugs as a way of coping with the problem. Remind the patient that using substances only aggravates the situation.

• Check for the presence or worsening of symptoms such as significant impairment in functioning.

• Clarify treatment compliance.

• Ask for support from family members. Some patients prefer to be in the company of caring people during these difficult times.

• Encourage the patient to see a physician or mental health professionals.

• Avoid arguments, confrontations, and criticisms. This is not the best time to engage in fruitless communication.

• Tell the patient to delay making major decisions while sick, such as resigning from a job.

• Build the patient's hopes. Share your own experiences or the experiences of others in successfully dealing with the illness. Remind the patient that current difficulties are just temporary. If the patient has an appointment with a health care professional, reassure him/her that help is coming.

• Appreciate the patient's positive comments about self. Correct the patient's low opinion of himself/herself. Avoid putting down the patient.

• Help the patient apply for sick or emergency leave.

- Help the patient organize daily activities and routine. Assist patients who lack the motivation to establish structure by writing to-do lists and making appointments.

- Allow the person to talk and share emotions, concerns, and issues at a certain time of the day.

- Appreciate patients' efforts to help themselves such as through improved nutrition and sleep, and participation in activities.

Chapter 15

Psychosis

Case Scenario

Mr. U, a 19-year-old college student, was observed to have "changed a lot" by his classmates. He was known to be neat and well dressed and he never missed a day of school. For the past seven months however, he attended class irregularly and when he did attend, he appeared untidy, malodorous, and unshaved. He was also observed to be "somewhat preoccupied" in class, occasionally mumbling to himself. His concerned instructor referred him to the school counselor for evaluation.

Mr. U reported that he had been hearing "voices" for the past year. He said that the "voices," coming from both men and women, had told him how bad he was, and that he was a "faggot." He described the voices as coming from outside his head, as occurring on and off during the day, and as being very bothersome. He attempted to "do anything" such as listening to radio, or pacing back and forth, to make them go away. But they kept coming back. Moreover, a few months ago, he began to receive messages from the television. He said that the "special" messages were picked up by a microchip embedded in his chin. When asked about the messages, he stated that they were messages coming from God to him –"God's beloved son."

How is psychosis manifested?

Patients suffering from psychosis develop a variety of symptoms. Hallucinations are common. When patients experience auditory hallucination, they complain of hearing sounds or voices that others cannot hear. These sounds are described as buzzing, musical, knocking on the door, or footsteps in the hallway. When they hear "voices," they describe them as if someone is talking to them. Some patients describe the voices as clear while others report an inaudible or mumbling voice. Some describe hearing only one voice while others hear multiple voices from both men and women. Those who hear the voices audibly sometimes describe them as critical of them, telling them how bad they are, that they deserve the damnation of hell, and that they will not amount to anything. Some people, however, describe nice and pleasant voices such as voices singing church hymns.

Visual hallucination occasionally occurs along with the auditory hallucination. Patients complain of seeing things such as a person, object, or animals, which others cannot see. A patient may complain of seeing rats running around the room and under the bed. Occasionally, gustatory (referring to taste) hallucination happens. At this time, patients describe a particular taste that is not experienced by others. Some patients experience olfactory hallucination – smelling something like a burning tire – that others cannot smell.

As mentioned in Chapter 8, delusions are inappropriate ideas or beliefs that patients hold strongly. Patients develop thoughts that are unusual and not typically held by people of the same ethnic group and culture. There are many types of delusion. Patients with bizarre delusions experience thought broadcasting, that is, they believe that others hear their thoughts or that their thoughts are broadcasted to everyone. Delusions of mind reading occur when patients develop the belief that others can read their mind, or that they can actually read other people's minds. Other forms of bizarre delusion include thought insertion and thought withdrawal. Thought insertion occurs when patients believe that others insert ideas in their mind. Thought withdrawal occurs when patients believe that their thoughts are actually taken from their mind by others.

Some patients suffer from persecutory delusion. This is exhibited when they develop the belief that people are after them, that someone is laughing at them, that their neighbors are conspiring to assassinate them, that their phones are bugged, or that their co-workers follow them. Other patients develop delusions of reference. In this case, they believe that the actors and actresses on the television, the newscaster or the music on the radio are referring to them and sending them special messages. Delusions of grandeur also occur. Patients believe that they are the messiah, the last prophet, or the son of God; or that they have supernatural abilities; or that the US President or the Prime Minister of Canada consults them in policy decisions.

Some patients with psychosis develop thought disorganization in which they tend to jump from one topic to another one which is logically unrelated. A patient, for example, who is talking about his mother suddenly changes the topic to the weather. Some patients have a tangential thought process, in which their answers are not logically connected to questions asked of them. Patients with severe thought disorganization are generally very difficult to understand.

Some patients show thought blocking and are unable to sustain the flow of thought. They stop unnecessarily, for example, when talking about their mother. Still others develop bizarre mannerisms such as maintaining a certain posture or hand position; or echolalia and echopraxia, which refer to imitating the last words or actions respectively of the person talking to them.

Along with the above symptoms, the patients gradually develop impairment in functioning. They have difficulty at work or school, and they cannot function at home or perform their usual activities. Even doing household chores become a struggle. Some patients withdraw from social situations, preferring to be on their own without contact with anyone.

Case scenario

Mr. U further deteriorated after he threw in the garbage the medication prescribed for him. He figured he didn't need the medication anyway since he was "not really sick." He completely stopped going to school. His apartment was dirty and malodorous due to spoiled food. Subsequently, his landlord evicted him for his failure to pay the rent and keep the place clean. He ended up living on the street, rummaging for food at night. With poor nutrition and no housing, he developed health problems.

One day, while in the subway station, the "voices" told him to push an elderly man on to the ramp of an approaching train. The chip in his chin had received a message from the train about the "plan." The next day he was in the newspaper headlines.

What are the complications to anticipate?

Significant functional impairment eventually ensues. Patients cannot go to work anymore, clean the house, and take care of physical health. They also abandon personal hygiene so that medical problems such as electrolyte imbalance and infection are common. Unemployed, some patients become homeless, staying on the streets regardless of weather conditions which compounds their medical problems. Patients often develop poor judgment and lack of understanding as a result of the illness. Moreover, an inability to control impulses becomes an issue. Patients engage in violent behavior especially when they are severely paranoid or delusional. A young patient who thought that she was the messiah killed another person as a "sacrifice to save the world." Some psychotic patients become suicidal. One patient hung himself in the bedroom, perhaps as a way to "escape," because he thought that his neighbor was out to get him.

What illnesses manifest psychosis?

Several primary psychiatric disorders, excessive alcohol and substance use, and medical conditions can cause psychosis.

Schizophrenia

Schizophrenia is a chronic illness characterized by impairment in thought and behavior. Hallucinations, paranoia, and bizarre delusions are typical symptoms. Certain features such as disorganized behavior, blunted to flat affect, withdrawn state, lack of motivation, and gradual deterioration of functioning also appear. The symptoms ordinarily develop in the late teens to early twenties and usually last more than six months. The onset is earlier among men. This illness has about a 1% risk of developing in a lifetime.

Schizophrenia has a strong genetic component as shown by studies on twins. However, biological factors, such as neurotransmitter changes (dopamine, serotonin, norepinephrine, and amino acid), widening of the third and lateral ventricles of the brain, and abnormalities in the basal ganglia, have also been implicated.

As mentioned above, the illness starts in the adolescent period and it may be precipitated by stressors. Gradual impairment of functioning and isolation develop. Depression that occurs after an acute episode increases likelihood of disability and suicide risk. Although about 50% frequently experience a relapse with the illness, about 25% may be able to live normal lives. Treatment includes medications, psychotherapy, provision of shelter and food, rehabilitation, and day programs.

DSM-IV Diagnostic Criteria for Schizophrenia

A. Characteristic symptoms: Two (or more) of the following, each present for a significant portion of time during a 1-month period (or less if successfully treated):
    1) delusions
    2) hallucinations

3) disorganized speech
4) grossly disorganized or catatonic behavior
5) negative symptoms, i.e., affective flattening, alogia, or avolition

Note: Only one Criterion A symptom is required if delusions are bizarre or hallucinations consist of a voice keeping up a running commentary on the person's behavior or thoughts, or two or more voices conversing with each other.

B. Social/occupational dysfunction: For a significant portion of the time since the onset of the disturbance, one or more major areas of functioning such as work, interpersonal relations, or self-care are markedly below the level achieved prior to the onset.

C. Duration: Continuous signs of the disturbance persist for at least 6 months. This 6-month period must include at least 1 month of symptoms (or less if successfully treated) that meet Criterion A (i.e., active-phase symptoms) and may include periods of prodromal or residual symptoms. During these prodromal or residual periods, the signs of the disturbance may be manifested by only negative symptoms or two or more symptoms listed in Criterion A present in an attenuated form (e.g., odd beliefs, unusual perceptual experiences).

D. Schizoaffective and Mood Disorder exclusion: Schizoaffective Disorder and Mood Disorder with Psychotic features have been ruled out because either 1) no Major Depressive, Manic, or Mixed Episodes have occurred concurrently with the active-phase symptoms; or 2) if mood episodes have occurred during active-phase symptoms, their total duration has been brief relative to the duration of the active and residual periods.

E. Substance/general medical condition exclusion: The disturbance is not due to the direct physiological effects of a substance or a general medical condition.

F. Relationship to Pervasive Developmental Disorder: If there is a history of Autistic Disorder or another Pervasive Developmental Disorder, the additional diagnosis of Schizophrenia is made only if prominent delusions or hallucinations are also present for at least a month.

Reprinted with permission from the Diagnostic and Statistical Manual of Mental Disorders, Fourth Edition, Text Revision. Copyright 2000 American Psychiatric Association.

Brief Psychotic Disorder

Brief psychotic disorder presents with the same symptoms as schizophrenia, but the duration is less than one month. Usually this illness is preceded by a stressor, such as separation or divorce, and appears suddenly in people with premorbid personality disorder and in those belonging to a low socioeconomic class. A common presentation among patients is disorganized speech associated with mood instability or inattention.

The etiology is unclear. Relatives of patients have a higher risk of developing mood disorder. Prognosis is generally good. Treatment includes antipsychotic medications and psychotherapy.

Schizophreniform Disorder

Schizophreniform disorder presents with the same symptoms as schizophrenia or brief psychotic disorder but the duration of the illness is at least one month and less than six months. It has a 0.2% risk of developing in a lifetime. The etiology is unknown but brain imaging has shown widening or enlargement of the ventricles in the brain. This illness has a better prognosis than schizophrenia. Treatment includes use of antipsychotic medications and psychotherapy.

Schizoaffective Disorder

Schizoaffective disorder is a chronic illness characterized by schizophrenia symptoms along with a substantial impairment in mood, either depression or mania. The disorder has less than a 1% chance of developing in a lifetime and is more prevalent among women. Its etiology is currently unclear. It has a better prognosis than schizophrenia but has a worse prognosis than a mood disorder. Treatment includes antipsychotic medications and mood stabilizers as well as psychosocial programs.

Delusional Disorder

Delusional disorder is an illness that has delusion as its predominant symptom. In this illness, the delusion is considered "non-bizarre" that is, the inappropriate beliefs can be based on actual or possible situations. Some delusions include beliefs that a celebrity is madly in love with the affected person, that someone is out to get him or her, or that the spouse is having an affair. Other areas of the patient's life are not significantly affected by the illness. Hallucination is rare or non-existent. The illness has a 0.03% chance of developing in a lifetime. It is more common among women than men, and those affected are mostly married and employed.

The etiology is unknown but relatives of delusional patients have an increased likelihood to develop delusional disorder, schizophrenia, or mood disorder. Stressors may precipitate the onset of the illness. Of those affected, about 50% recover. The prognosis is generally good for patients whose illness develops before age thirty, is of sudden onset and of short duration. Treatment includes antipsychotic medications and psychotherapy.

Psychotic Disorder Due to General Medical Condition/ Substance-induced Psychotic Disorder

Some medical conditions that can cause psychosis include brain tumor, systemic lupus erythematosus, neurosyphilis, and Vitamin B-12 deficiency. Substances, especially illicit ones, can also cause psychosis. These substances include alcohol, LSD, cocaine, PCP, mescaline, ketamine, steroids, amphetamines, and thyroxin.

Other Conditions Manifesting With Psychosis

A number of mental illnesses such as personality disorder, dementia, major depressive disorder, bipolar disorder, and other major psychiatric disorder can also present with psychosis.

Early intervention

For Patients:
- Apply the HEAL technique.

- Accept the signs and symptoms of psychosis and deal with them.

- Reduce stress by recognizing and addressing problems and issues including possible triggers or precipitants.
Example:
> Financial concerns especially with respect to medication represent a big problem for psychotic patients. If you experience this problem, approach government agencies and seek financial and medical assistance.

- Socialize with friends and close relatives.

- Try to cope with hallucinations by listening to the radio, participating in physical activity, talking to people, and changing body positions.

- For delusions, apply thought restructuring especially in dealing with paranoia or suspiciousness. Verify conclusions about certain individuals, and consider alternative explanations of others' motives.

- Learn problem-solving skills.
Example:
> You realize that drinking alcohol has made you worse. However, your drinking friends keep inviting you to hang out with them. You decide to stop drinking and you think of ways to tell your friends politely about your decision. After much thought, you choose to tell them about your condition and your reason for not drinking.

- Comply with treatment and medication recommended by the physician.

- Check for the presence or worsening of symptoms, such as distressing hallucinations and delusions, inability to function, and disheveled appearance.

- Communicate needs, such as housing and financial support, to your health care worker or government agencies.

- Avoid using mood-altering substances such as alcohol and other illicit drugs. Using substances can only aggravate the situation.

- Check for early presence of hallucinations and delusions.

- Ask a hospital emergency room, crisis line, or mental health services for help.

- Check for the presence of medication side effects such as tremors and involuntary movements of the face and mouth.

- Cope with suicidal or homicidal thoughts via diversion: physical diversion includes recreational activities and exercise; social diversion includes going out and visiting friends and relatives; mental diversion involves replacement of the predominant thought. Informing someone and talking about suicidal or homicidal thoughts to close friends and relatives are beneficial in prevention.

- Deal with anger through anger management.

- For sleep problems, apply sleep hygiene.

- Deal with anxiety through the use of relaxation techniques such as breathing exercises and progressive muscle relaxation.

- Identify activities that make you feel better.

- Organize daily activities and routine.

- Ask for support from family members. Some relatives are willing to share their time and resources to help people in need.

- Deal with inappropriate thoughts through thought restructuring.

- Delay making major decisions while sick. Many people can't make rational choices when their minds are impaired by the illness.

- Establish realistic and achievable goals.

- Renew or strengthen your spirituality. Being connected with the higher power offers hope, inner confidence, guidance, and comfort.

For Caregivers:

- Apply the HELP method.

- Accept the patient's on-going signs and symptoms of psychosis. Consider them as manifestations of an illness that must be addressed.

- Administer the medication prescribed by the physician (if patient is unable to) or encourage medication self-management.

- Avoid arguments, confrontations, and criticisms. Help in minimizing distress in the family.

- Check for the early presence of hallucinations and delusions such as talking to oneself, isolation, and inappropriate fears and beliefs.

- Ask about the presence of medication side effects such as tremors, weight gain, constipation, and involuntary movements of the face or mouth.

- Clarify safety by asking about the presence of suicidal or homicidal thoughts.

- Be alert for signs of threat to self or self-destructive behavior such as superficial cuts on the wrist, compliance with command hallucination, goodbye letters, giving away possessions, taking a gun out of the cabinet, and unprovoked agitation and violence. Be alert for any agitated or aggressive behavior as shown by pacing back and forth, easily getting upset for no reason, and becoming verbally abusive.

- Encourage the avoidance of mood-altering substances such as alcohol and other illicit drugs as a way of coping with the problem. Remind the patient that using substances only aggravates the situation.

- Check for worsening of symptoms, such as disheveled appearance, bizarre behavior, and inability to function.

- Call for help to a hospital emergency room, crisis line, and police officers if there is an imminent danger to oneself or others, or an inability to take care of oneself.

- Clarify treatment compliance. Ask the patient if he/she has been taking the medications prescribed by the physician.

- Communicate needs, such as housing and financial support, to government agencies.

- Contain aggressive and violent behavior by locking the doors and keeping weapons away. Try your best to keep the patient and yourself safe.

- Teach the patient some problem-solving skills. Ask patients to weigh the benefits and risks of their decisions.

- Encourage socialization.

- Attend to the patient's personal hygiene and medical needs.

- Help in addressing housing concerns.

- Assist in recognizing and addressing problems and issues including possible triggers or precipitants.

- Help the patient cope with the hallucinations and delusions by some practical interventions.

- Encourage the patient to establish goals.

Chapter **16**

Excessive Drug or Alcohol Use

Case Scenario

Ms. T is a 44-year-old divorced, unemployed female who was referred for further evaluation and treatment. Ms. T started drinking alcohol at age sixteen while at a prom. At first, she did not like the taste of liquor but after drinking binges with friends on weekends, "just for the fun of it," she began to crave it. Before she knew it, she was drinking regularly. At age 25, she drank alcohol almost daily – a liter of vodka and several cans of beer. She used to drink almost immediately after she woke up. She realized she couldn't do without alcohol even for a day. Without it, she would experience anxiety, sweating, headache, and tremulousness.

Subsequently, her excessive drinking resulted in absences at work and an inability to perform assigned tasks. She also failed to take care of herself, especially her hygiene and appearance. After she lost her job, she had more free time, most of which was spent drinking. She began to neglect her three young kids. Despite all this, she never realized the alcohol's negative impact on her life. Her husband hated the changes he saw in her, and he gradually became withdrawn and resigned to her fate. He never bothered to seek help for her. He later sought a divorce since he could no longer tolerate her behavior and the constant smell of alcohol in the household.

How is alcohol/drug abuse or dependence manifested?

Heavy use of illicit drugs or alcohol is common. Some patients use a substantial amount of alcohol or substances daily, such as more than a dozen beer or more than a gram of marijuana per day. The majority of abusing or dependent patients have had long periods of repeated use – more than three years. They badly crave the substance and have a lot of difficulty if they cannot obtain and use the substance when they need it. It is common for them to develop a tolerance for the substance, that is, they feel the need to increase the intake after each use to get the same effect. Patients who have used the substance for a significant period have experienced withdrawal signs and symptoms after they suddenly stop usage. Such a withdrawal state consists of a variety of physical and emotional changes. Sudden discontinuation of alcohol, for example, may result in tremors, sweating, anxiety, irritability, palpitations, and headache, while stopping heroin use can result in generalized pain, loose bowel movement, runny nose, goose pimples, and yawning.

Due to their preoccupation with the substance, they begin to neglect personal hygiene and appearance. Long-term use takes its toll on their bodies, resulting in various medical problems such as liver cirrhosis, hepatitis, and HIV (through sharing of needles). They are also unable to function normally at work, school, or even at home. They frequently miss work, to the dismay of their employer and co-workers. Also, academic and other worthwhile pursuits are put aside in favor of using the substance or hanging around with people who use them. At home, cleanliness and basic chores are ignored.

Case scenario

Ms. T continued to drink despite the advice from close family and friends. She drank more and more to experience a feeling of "well-being." Preoccupied with alcohol, she was unable to attend to her basic needs including proper eating, bathing, and other health habits. She rarely left her house. If she did go out, it was to buy more alcoholic beverages. Since she had already lost her driver's license a few years earlier because of repetitive drinking and driving violations, she would walk to the liquor store even in the coldest part of winter.

As time passed, Ms. T's situation got worse. One day she suddenly woke up with severe tremors, sweating, and hallucinations. She saw small "animals" running around under the table and sofa and crawling on the wall. A concerned neighbor, who had not seen her outside her house for a few days, entered her house and saw her lying down on the floor looking "confused." She was rushed to the hospital. At the emergency room, it was noted that she lost a lot of weight and had a vitamin deficiency. Further tests revealed an enlarged liver.

What are the complications to anticipate?

Heavy alcohol and drug use has deleterious consequences. Many patients who use substances encounter legal troubles such as drinking while intoxicated, reckless driving, assault, drug pushing and possession, armed robbery, breaking and entering, and the like.

Some lose their savings and employment and become involved in criminal activities and prostitution in order to sustain their use. Suicidal behavior may occur if there is associated mood instability such as depression. Violence and homicide can happen because chronic use impairs judgment. Medical problems are common when there is prolonged use. If drugs or alcohol use is suddenly stopped, patients may experience withdrawal signs and symptoms. Delirium tremens, a condition which exhibits hallucination, disorientation, inattention, drowsiness and other withdrawal signs and symptoms, may occur.

Tolerance or the need to increase the dose of intake to obtain a euphoric effect, and dependence, a psychological or physiologic state associated with the need to use a substance to achieve a desired effect or "to avoid the discomfort of its absence" (Dorland's, 1994), occur among chronic and heavy users. Significant impairment in functioning occurs when patients spend a lot of time acquiring and using the substance. Some also develop auditory hallucinations, depression, anxiety, and paranoia as a result of either intake or withdrawal from a substance. Spouses and children are neglected. Given these realities, many patients develop conflict and other relational problems with their spouses, children, and close relatives. Furthermore, death may result from vehicle-related accidents, violence, and medical problems such as liver cirrhosis and cancer.

What are the common drugs associated with abuse and dependence?

Cannabis

Marijuana is the most commonly used form of Cannabis. The drug results in euphoria in less than an hour and it can be smoked or taken orally with food. Physical effects of the drug, such as eye redness and dryness of mouth, are observable several minutes after use. Users sometimes have accidents involving vehicles or machinery. Medical problems such as bronchitis are not unusual. Infants (breastfeeding babies) of mothers using cannabis may suffer weight loss. Mental conditions, such as psychosis, delirium, lack of motivation, and anxiety, have also been reported. Psychological dependence, or craving the drug, occurs especially among chronic users. When long-term users suddenly stop using the drug, they experience subtle withdrawal symptoms, as manifested by agitation, mood instability, and inability to sleep. Treatment includes detoxification, abstinence, counseling, rehabilitation, and psychoeducation.

Cocaine, amphetamines and other stimulants

Amphetamines consist of dextroamphetamine methylphenidate, ephedrine and phenylpropranolamine. This type of drug can be taken orally or intravenously. With intravenous use, the onset of action is rapid resulting in euphoria through release of neurotransmitters, such as serotonin, dopamine and norepinephrine. The users of this drug are usually in their late teens or early adulthood. Treatment includes detoxification, abstinence, counseling, psychoeducation, rehabilitation, and group therapy.

Cocaine is known to be highly addictive. Crack is a potent preparation of this drug and it is commonly used by late teens and young adults. Snorting, injection, smoking, and inhalation are methods of drug usage with smoking and intravenous injection considered unsafe routes of introduction. This drug increases the neurotransmitters (such as dopamine, serotonin, and norepinephrine) in the brain by blocking their reuptake to the presynaptic cell. Its onset of action and resulting euphoria occur rapidly.

Complications occur. Medical problems are common, such as seizure, chorea (dance-like type of abnormal movements), brain infarction and hemorrhage, arrhythmias (irregular heart beats) and other heart concerns, HIV, hypertension, and fetal death or abnormalities in pregnancy. Death may even ensue if the medical complications become severe and uncontrollable. As with heroin, suicidal and violent behavior, criminal activities, and death may happen. Suicidal thoughts occur when patients become very depressed, especially after suddenly stopping cocaine use. Intoxication or taking high doses of cocaine at one time can result in physiologic changes, such as increase in heart rate, sweating, high blood pressure, behavioral changes, mood instability and difficulty controlling one's impulses. Emotional changes, such as psychosis, depression, euphoria, and anxiety, may also appear. Tolerance, dependence, and withdrawal signs and symptoms ensue among chronic and heavy users. Treatment should include detoxification, abstinence, counseling, psychoeducation, rehabilitation, and group therapy.

Opiates or Heroin

Heroin and other opioids, such as morphine, codeine, and hydromorphone have almost the same properties. They affect the opioid receptor and other neurotransmitters, such as serotonin and dopamine, in the brain. This type of receptor is responsible for dependence. The use of this drug usually occurs in the early teens. Heroin is abused more frequently than other opioids. More men are heavy users of opioids than women. Several factors have been implicated as the possible cause. Heavy use of opioids is common among those with a low socioeconomic status. A strong genetic component is also possible.

Various complications are common. Given the increased potential for heroin users to have medical problems and be involved in criminal activities such as drug pushing and possession, death can occur. Patients develop suicidal and violent behavior. Several medical conditions become prominent such as HIV infection (especially for those who share needles), subacute bacterial endocarditis (heart infection), bacteremia (infection in the blood), tetanus, pulmonary emboli (lung problem), transverse myelitis (spinal cord disease), polyneuropathy (nerve problems), and renal failure. Mood changes and psychosis may also appear during the course of heroin use. Tolerance, dependence, and withdrawal signs and symptoms ensue among chronic and heavy users. Treatment includes substitution with methadone or LAAM or abstinence after detoxification, psychoeducation, counseling, rehabilitation, and group therapy.

Alcohol

Heavy alcohol use is the third largest health problem in the United States. Increased mortality among heavy alcohol users is due to homicide, suicide, medical problems, and accidents. Alcohol use along with clinical depression increases the risk of suicide. Heavy use is more common among men than women. Studies on twins and adoptees have shown a strong genetic component for this type of illness. Alcohol, when taken in combination with other sedative-hypnotic drugs such as barbiturates, benzodiazepine, and antidepressants can be dangerous because of resulting complications, such as stupor or coma. Heavy alcohol use has numerous deleterious consequences. Legal troubles such as driving while intoxicated and assault may ensue. Suicidal and violent behavior are common. Medical problems associated with heavy alcohol use include fetal malformation from drinking during pregnancy, coma, dementia, head trauma, thiamine deficiency, cirrhosis, gastritis, aspiration pneumonia, pancreatitis, electrolyte imbalance, cancer, cardiomyopathy, and cerebrovascular disease. Delirium tremens may occur. Patients who have taken alcohol for many years experience blackouts, that is, an inability to remember "new" events after the drinking episode. Some also develop auditory hallucinations and paranoia. Tolerance and dependence appear in chronic and heavy users. Substantial impairment in functioning is a typical result. Furthermore, death may result from vehicle-related accidents and from medical problems, such as liver cirrhosis and cancer. Treatment includes detoxification, abstinence, psychotherapy, counseling, AA, rehabilitation and group therapies.

Sedative-Hypnotic-Anxiolytic Drugs

These drugs, mostly given by restricted prescription, have roughly the same broad effects as alcohol. They include benzodiazepines, such as lorazepam and alprazolam; and barbiturates, such as phenobarbital and barbiturate-like substances like methaqualone. They inhibit the GABA receptors in the brain. Like alcohol, they cause tolerance and psychological and physical dependence. Double doctoring is common among users. Dependence on this type of drug is more common among women than men. While benzodiazepines are tolerable on overdose, barbiturate overdose is dangerous and may be fatal. Treatment includes detoxification, abstinence, rehabilitation, counseling, and psychotherapy.

Phencyclidine or PCP

PCP, also known as angel dust or crystal, has an anesthetic effect. It is known to be an NMDA (N-methyl-D-aspartate) antagonist. It significantly affects the dopaminergic system resulting in euphoria and physical effects such as increase in heart rate and blood pressure. After intake, effects occur in a few hours and last for several days. Men use the drug more than women. Most users belong to the 20 to 40 year old range.

Heavy PCP use gives rise to various problems such as hallucinations and confusion. Medical complications associated with its use include renal failure, hypertension, and hyperthermia (high body temperature), and at very high dosages, coma and even death are possible. Socially inappropriate behavior includes disrobing in public and masturbating in the presence of others. Aggressive tendencies are most likely among chronic users. In time, tolerance and psychological and physical dependence also appear. Treatment includes detoxification, abstinence, counseling, psychotherapy, and rehabilitation.

LSD

LSD develops its effects within sixty minutes of intake but the peak effect occurs in about three hours. The drug acts as a partial agonist at the postsynaptic serotonin receptor. The route of use includes inhalation, smoking, oral intake, and intravenous injection. This drug causes perceptual changes. Some users, for example, perceive the color of the wall as brighter and the rose smelling nicer. Visual hallucinations, especially regarding shapes and forms of objects, are common. The individual's mood becomes unpredictable and unstable. At times, users may be euphoric and at other times, depressed. Heavy use of LSD is more common among men than women. Individuals of ages 15 to 35 are the most common users.

LSD is known to cause hallucinations, especially visual and manic-like symptoms, at high doses. Cerebrovascular disease and death may result if taken indiscriminately. Although tolerance and psychological dependence occur, physical dependence is not found even among heavy LSD users.

DSM-IV Diagnostic Criteria for Substance Dependence

A maladaptive patterns of substance use, leading to clinically significant impairment or distress, as manifested by three (or more) of the following, occurring at any time in the same 12-month period:
1) tolerance, as defined by either of the following:
    a) a need for markedly increased amounts of the substance to achieve intoxication or desired effect
    b) markedly diminished effect with continued use of the same amount of the substance
2) withdrawal, as manifested by either of the following:
    a) the characteristic withdrawal syndrome for the substance
    b) the same (or a closely related) substance is taken to relieve or avoid withdrawal symptoms
3) the substance is often taken in larger amounts or over a longer period than was intended
4) there is a persistent desire or successful efforts to cut down or control substance use
5) a great deal of time is spent in activities necessary to obtain the substance, use the substance, or recover from its effects
6) important social, occupational, or recreational activities are given up or reduced because of substance use
7) the substance use is continued despite knowledge of having a persistent or recurrent physical or psychological problem that is likely to have been caused or exacerbated by the substance

DSM-IV Diagnostic Criteria for Substance Abuse

A. A maladaptive pattern of substance use leading to clinically significant impairment or distress, as manifested by one (or more) of the following, occurring within a 12-month period:
    1) recurrent substance use resulting in a failure to fulfill major role obligations at work, school, or home
    2) recurrent substance in situations in which it is physically hazardous
    3) recurrent substance-related legal problems
    4) continued substance use despite having persistent or recurrent social or interpersonal problems caused or exacerbated by the effects of the substance
B. The symptoms have never met the criteria for Substance dependence for this class of substance.

Both criteria are reprinted with permission from the Diagnostic and Statistical Manual of Mental Disorders, Fourth Edition, Text Revision. Copyright 2000 American Psychiatric Association.

Early intervention

For patients:
- Apply the HEAL technique.

- Accept the signs and symptoms of abuse or dependence and deal with them.

- Establish friendship with non-users.

- Cultivate lasting healthy relationships.

- Seek support through self-help groups such as Alcoholics Anonymous (AA), Narcotics Anonymous (NA) or Cocaine Anonymous (CA).

- Pursue new goals, interests, and experiences.

- Recognize the causes of craving. Avoid bars and nightclubs.

- Develop coping strategies to reduce craving, such as through diversion.

Example:
> Each time you experience a craving for drugs, choose to keep yourself busy, to perform a chore, or to involve yourself in physical activities.

- Cut off ties with the source of illicit drugs.

- Undergo counseling, detoxification, and rehabilitation programs.

- Learn to socialize without having to resort to drugs or alcohol.

- Learn to effectively express needs and feelings.

- Assess the negative impact of substance use on your life.

- Attend to your physical health.

- Deal with anxiety through relaxation techniques such as breathing exercises and progressive muscle relaxation.

- Deal with anger through anger management.

- For sleep problems, apply sleep hygiene.

- For patients with low self-esteem, practice self-affirmation. Write in a notebook or journal a least three good things about yourself daily. These positive comments should be reviewed frequently. Dwell on positive experiences in the present and the past. Read literature that uplifts the spirit.

- Identify activities that make you feel better.

- Cope with suicidal or homicidal thoughts via diversion: physical diversion includes recreational activities and exercise; social diversion includes going out and visiting friends and relatives; mental diversion involves replacement of the predominant thought. Informing someone and talking about suicidal or homicidal thoughts to close friends and relatives are beneficial in prevention.

- Reduce stress by recognizing and addressing problems and issues, including possible triggers or precipitants.

• Comply with the treatment and medication as recommended by the physician.

• Check for the presence or worsening of symptoms such as excessive drinking and drugging, and significant impairment in functioning.

• Organize schedule of daily activities and routine.

• Ask for support from family members. Some relatives are willing to share their time and resources to help people in need.

• Ask for help and do not hesitate to call a hospital emergency room, crisis line, or mental health/addiction services. Seek an assessment by an addiction specialist.

• Delay making major decisions while sick, such as selling the house, stealing, engaging in prostitution to maintain the habit. Many people can't make rational choices when substance use impairs the mind.

• Weigh the benefits and risks of abuse and dependence.

• Renew or strengthen your spirituality. Being connected with the higher power offers hope, inner confidence, guidance, and comfort.

For caregivers:
• Apply the HELP technique.

• Accept the signs and symptoms of abuse or dependence and deal with them. Consider them as manifestations of an illness that must be addressed.

• Recognize scenarios that place patients at high-risk for relapse and discuss them with patients. Assess family factors that contribute to the problem and provide some solutions.

• Encourage the patient to attend self-help programs such as Alcoholics Anonymous (AA), Narcotics Anonymous (NA), or Cocaine Anonymous (CA).

• Monitor the patient for high-risk or self-destructive behavior, suicidality, homicidality, and violence.

- For intoxicated individuals, minimize noise and other forms of stimulation.

- Appreciate sobriety and efforts to remain "clean" from substances.

- Listen to the patient's concerns and issues.

- Discuss with individuals the negative impact of substance use on their lives.

- Discourage major changes in the patient's life. Encourage the patient to delay major decisions, such as divorce or resigning from a job, while still sick.

- Administer the medication prescribed by the physician (if the patient is unable to) or encourage medication self-management.

- Avoid arguments, confrontations, and criticisms.

- Clarify safety by asking about the presence of suicidal or homicidal thoughts.

- Be alert for signs of threat to self or self-destructive behavior such as superficial cuts on the wrist, goodbye letters, giving away possessions, taking a gun out of the cabinet. Be alert for any agitated or aggressive behavior as shown by pacing back and forth, easily getting upset for no reason, becoming verbally abusive, and exhibiting unprovoked agitation and violence.

- Encourage the avoidance of mood-altering substances such as alcohol and other illicit drugs as a way of coping with the problem. Remind the patient that using substances only aggravates the situation.

- Check for the early presence of emotional difficulties, such as hallucinations, delusions, anxiety, and depression.

- Check for worsening of symptoms, for example disheveled appearance and inability to function.

- Call for help from a hospital emergency room, crisis line, or police officers if there is an imminent danger to self or others, inability to take care of self, and serious medical problems.

• Clarify treatment compliance. Ask patients if they have been taking the medications prescribed by the physician.

• Teach the patient some problem-solving skills (as described in Chapter 7).

• Help minimize distress in the family.

• Encourage socialization.

• Attend to the patient's personal hygiene and medical needs.

• Assist in recognizing and addressing problems and issues, including possible triggers or precipitants.

• Help the patient cope with intense craving via behavioral intervention which includes physical exercise, hobbies, or artistic endeavors.

• Allow patients to learn from their mistakes and be accountable for their actions. For instance, do not bail them out if they get into legal trouble (drinking and driving, assault, or robbery) in using and acquiring the substance.

• Seek help from support groups such as Al-anon and Adult Children of Alcoholics.

Chapter **17**

Eating Disorder

Case Scenario

Ms. P is a 16-year-old high school student referred by the school counselor due to concerns about her weight. According to the report, Ms. P had lost a significant amount of weight over the past six months. Her close friends and classmates disclosed to the counselor her "secret" activities to lose weight, such as self-induced vomiting, excessive exercise, and occasionally, the use of over-the-counter anti-constipation medication. Ms. P is 5'8" tall but weighs 87 pounds.

Ms. P's preoccupation with weight started when classmates began to talk about models, actresses, and singers. Although all were interested in maintaining a "pretty body," nobody had matched Ms. P's fascination with thinness and body image.

Believing she was "too fat," Ms. P became involved in a rigorous exercise regimen using a treadmill. She began to monitor her caloric intake. She developed a plan to "diet" by eating only a few cookies for a meal. After eating, she would go to the washroom to induce herself to vomit. Before long, she became very thin. Her parents had noticed the change but she tried to hide her thin appearance by wearing loose and padded clothing. Despite her weight loss, Ms. P still believed she was "fat."

How is the illness manifested?

Preoccupation with weight and apprehension about caloric intake are common among patients with an eating disorder. They develop an obsessional preoccupation with weight so that they closely monitor the number of calories they ingest and the food they eat. They try to hide food and lie about food intake. Efforts to lose weight by any means are attempted. Some patients induce vomiting after every meal, some use laxatives and others use diuretics or medications that cause passage of urine. In order to lose weight or to prevent weight gain, patients turn to excessive exercise and fasting. One female patient exercised at least two hours per day just to burn off calories, and she tried hard to avoid food, eating just one spoonful of cereal. Patients also engage in binge eating in which they eat a large amount of high-caloric food such as cakes and other foods rich in carbohydrates. Generally patients harbor inappropriate thoughts about self-image and weight. They think and feel "fat" despite significant weight loss. They see themselves "bulging" in the mirror despite a cachectic appearance.

Case scenario

Ms. P maintained her rigid exercise regimen, self-induced vomiting, and fasting, and her physical health drastically deteriorated. One day she collapsed on the floor after she starved herself for three consecutive days. She ended up in the hospital where a complete work up, physical examination, and immediate medical intervention were done. She was noted to be extremely thin, with considerable electrolyte imbalance. Her heart rate was slow. Further evaluation revealed esophageal and heart problems. Had she not been treated in the hospital, her physicians felt that she could have died from the complications of the illness.

What are the complications to anticipate?

Medical problems are the major complications. Acute gastric dilatation, heart problems/cardiomyopathy, caries, gastroesophageal reflux, esophagitis, esophageal tears, and electrolyte imbalance may occur due to the induction of vomiting and the use of laxatives and diuretic medications. Patients who develop depression contemplate suicide.

Due to lack of food and fluid intake, starvation ensues. Once physical health falters, performing usual daily activities becomes increasingly difficult.

What illnesses manifest as eating disorder?

The two most common eating disorders are anorexia nervosa and bulimia nervosa. Medical conditions should be considered when significant weight loss is involved.

Anorexia Nervosa

Anorexia nervosa is a type of eating disorder in which the patients become involved in various weight-losing activities, such as excessive exercise, inappropriate use of laxatives or diuretics ("water pills"), self-induced vomiting and avoidance of food intake. Anorectic patients have an extreme "fear of gaining weight or becoming fat" (DSM IV). Despite substantial reductions in weight, they do not stop their inappropriate behavior. As a result, these patients develop medical problems. Medical complications noted include irregular heartbeats, inability to menstruate, extreme weight loss, electrolyte imbalance (e.g. low potassium), esophageal and gastric erosions, and seizures. The illness is common among women and usually develops in their midteens. About 4% of adolescents and young adults are afflicted with the illness.

A strong genetic component has been implicated as one of the possible causes, based on studies of twins. Brain imaging (CT SCAN) shows a widening of the brain's ventricles in some patients. Moreover, social factors have been implicated. Anorexia is more common in some professions, such as ballet and modeling. In general, the prognosis is poor with a mortality rate that ranges from 5 to 18%. The illness may co-exist with other illnesses such as major depressive disorder and dysthymic disorder. Treatment includes medical stabilization, if possible in a hospital setting. Behavioral and supportive therapy, psychoeducation, and medications such as selective serotonin reuptake inhibitor (SSRIs) may be tried. Hospitalization is necessary if a patient manifests substantial weight loss (> 30%), medical problems, suicidality and starvation.

DSM-IV Diagnostic Criteria for Anorexia Nervosa

A. Refusal to maintain body weight at or above a minimally normal weight for age and height (e.g., weight loss leading to maintenance of body weight less than 85% of that expected; or failure to make expected weight gain during period of growth, leading to body weight less than 85% of that expected).

B. Intense fear of gaining weight or becoming fat, even though underweight.

C. Disturbance in the way in which one's body weight or shape is experienced, undue influence of body weight or shape on self-evaluation, or denial of the seriousness of the current low body weight.

D. In postmenarcheal females, amenorrhea, i.e., the absence of at least three consecutive menstrual cycles.

Reprinted with permission from the Diagnostic and Statistical Manual of Mental Disorders, Fourth Edition, Text Revision. Copyright 2000 American Psychiatric Association.

Bulimia Nervosa

Bulimia nervosa is a type of illness that involves repetitive episodes of binge eating of sweets and high caloric foods, and inappropriate activities, such as self-induced vomiting, excessive exercise, or fasting, with the sole intention of preventing weight gain. In general, bulimic patients, unlike anorectic patients, maintain normal weight and remain sexually active. The illness may result in medical complications, such as electrolyte imbalance, esophageal and gastric erosion, and dental caries. The illness usually develops around late adolescence or early adulthood and has around a 1 to 3% risk of developing in a lifetime.

Some biological factors have been implicated. Neurotransmitters, such as serotonin and norepinephrine, may be affected. A genetic component is implicated by some studies which show that first-degree relatives have an increased risk of developing bulimia nervosa and mood disorder. The prognosis of bulimia nervosa is better than that of anorexia nervosa although medical problems may complicate the picture. About 50% of patients improve if treated appropriately. Recurrence may occur within five to ten years. Treatment includes medication, such as SSRIs, and behavioral and supportive therapy. Treatment may be given in the outpatient clinic. Hospitalization is indicated for a patient with worsening symptoms such as increasing binging and purging and medical complications.

DSM-IV Diagnostic Criteria for Bulimia Nervosa

A. Recurrent episodes of binge eating. An episode of binge eating is characterized by both of the following:

1) eating, in a discrete period of time (e.g., within any 2-hour period), an amount of food that is definitely larger than most people would eat during a similar period of time and under similar circumstances

2) a sense of lack of control over eating during the episode (e.g., a feeling that one cannot stop eating or control what or how much one is eating)

B. Recurrent inappropriate compensatory behavior in order to prevent weight gain, such as self-induced vomiting; misuse of laxatives, diuretics, enemas, or other medications; fasting; or excessive exercise.

C. The binge eating and inappropriate compensatory behaviors both occur, on average, at least twice a week for 3 months.

D. Self-evaluation is unduly influenced by body shape and weight.

E. The disturbance does not occur exclusively during episodes of Anorexia Nervosa.

Reprinted with permission from the Diagnostic and Statistical Manual of Mental Disorders, Fourth Edition, Text Revision. Copyright 2000 American Psychiatric Association.

Medical Conditions Presenting With Weight Loss

Medical problems that involve weight loss, such as tuberculosis, chron's disease, hyperthyroidism, and hypothalamic lesions, should be considered and ruled out before considering an illness as a primary eating disorder.

Early intervention

For Patients:

- Apply the HEAL technique.

- Accept binging, self-induced vomiting, fasting, and other signs and symptoms of eating disorder, and deal with them.

- Recognize and address the triggers of binging. By recognizing the cause, you may be able to create preventive measures. If a conflict with a co-worker precipitates your relapse, try to improve your work relationship through improved communication.

- Comply with the medication prescribed by your physician.

- Deal with anger and irritability through anger management.
Example:
> You constantly have an argument with your demanding mother. You realize that your relationship is "shaky." You decide that each time you begin to argue with your mom, you will avoid the situation by going to your bedroom or watch TV. After the anger has gone, try to communicate with your mother in a nice way.

- For sleep problem, apply sleep hygiene.

- Be alert for signs of threat to self or self-destructive behavior such as superficial cuts on the wrist, excessive exercise and use of diuretics and laxatives, serious medical complications, starvation, and substantial weight loss.

- Cope with suicidal thoughts through diversion: physical diversion involves activities such as recreational activities, going out, and exercise; social diversion includes visiting your friends and relatives; and mental diversion consists of mental activities such as thought replacement. Telling your relatives and therapist about thoughts of self-harm is beneficial in getting immediate help.

- Deal with anxiety through the use of relaxation techniques such as breathing exercises and progressive muscle relaxation.

- Deal with an inappropriate thought, such as that of being fat despite significant weight loss, by thought restructuring.
Example:
> Your weighing scale shows your weight as 80 lbs. Your height is 5'8". You feel fat despite a significant weight loss. Question yourself whether your actual weight is compatible with what you feel.

- If you have low self-esteem, practice self-affirmation. Write in a notebook or journal at least three good things about yourself daily. These positive comments need to be reviewed frequently. Also, dwell on positive experiences in the present and the past. Read positive literature that uplifts the spirit.

- Identify activities that make you feel better. If regular walks in the morning perks you up, then establish this routine.

- Call a hospital emergency room, crisis line, or mental health services for help.

- Ask for support from family members. Some relatives are willing to share their resources to help you solve your problem.

- Delay making major decisions while sick. The majority of people can't make rational choices when the mind is impaired by an illness.

- Organize daily activities and routine.

- Avoid putting yourself down. Don't blame yourself for the illness and the miseries of others.

- Avoid the use of mood-altering substances such as alcohol and other illicit drugs as a way of dealing with the illness. Using substances only adds to the problem.

- Immerse yourself in pleasant and positive thoughts. Negative and self-critical thoughts will make you feel worse.

- Strongly consider hospitalization when complications of the illness are observed.

- Renew or strengthen your spirituality. Being connected with the higher power offers hope, inner confidence, and comfort.

For Caregivers:

- Apply the HELP method.

- Accept the signs and symptoms of eating disorder. Consider them as manifestations of an illness that must be addressed.

- Monitor the patient's eating patterns, such as frequency of meals and type of food eaten.

- Check for inappropriate beliefs, such as thoughts of being fat despite significant weight loss.

- Be alert for signs of self-destructive behavior, such as excessive exercise, and the use of ipecac, laxatives, diuretics, and diet pills.

- Be aware of family interactions that may have contributed to the illness or that may have facilitated recovery.

- Check for inappropriate changes or behavior such as self-induced vomiting, binge eating, spontaneous vomiting, hiding food, food restriction and avoidances, ritualistic and compulsive behavior, or rapid loss of weight.

- Consider advising patient to see a nutritionist or a support group.

- Carefully plan meals and encourage food intake.

- Encourage seeing a family doctor for a check-up.

- Encourage the avoidance of mood-altering substances such as alcohol and other illicit drugs as a way of dealing with the illness.

- Monitor weight if possible.

- Reinforce patient's food intake through appreciation.

- Strongly consider hospitalizing the patient when you observe complications of the illness.

Chapter 18

Dementia or Memory Loss

Case Scenario

Ms. R is a 67-year-old former banker referred for evaluation by her family doctor due to "confusion." She reported having "forgetfulness for quite a while." She said that for the past several months, she had trouble remembering where she put things and could hardly remember phone numbers of her children. Her husband was upset that she forgot their 25th wedding anniversary. Despite such memory difficulties, Ms. R believed that forgetting "here and there" was part of normal aging. Her husband reported that her memory problems started about two years ago. At that time, she would look for her eyeglasses when in fact she was actually wearing them. She would forget names of familiar people such as neighbors and close friends. For the past two years, it was typical for her to ask, "Who was that person I was talking to?" when in fact she had known that person for years.

Her husband reported that she gradually got worse over the past six months. Occasionally, he had noticed her leaving the bathtub faucet on. On two occasions, she left the stove on after she cooked noodles. At night, she would question her husband about why he was there in the same bedroom as hers and would say, "I don't think my husband would like this." Her husband would remind her that he was her husband. She would then answer, "My husband is better looking than you!" Her husband, somewhat amused by the development, tolerated such confusion.

One day however, he received a call from the police about her. They said that Ms. R was driving around the mall, not knowing how to get out of the parking lot, and not knowing exactly how to get back home. They said that she appeared very "confused." She ended up in the emergency room for evaluation that day.

How is dementia manifested?

Dementia is manifested by persistent memory loss starting with recent events. Recent memory about food eaten for breakfast, activities done a few fours ago, and books and magazines read a day before, becomes problematic. Patients become forgetful about names of familiar people, important dates including doctors' appointment, anniversaries, and phone numbers of relatives. They also cannot name familiar objects such as a watch, pen, coat, or vase. Patients cannot remember where they keep and put things. Occasionally, they look for something, such as eyeglasses, a hat, or a watch, that they are actually wearing. Associated aphasia or language difficulty occurs. When this happens, patients develop trouble in understanding what they hear and difficulty in expressing what they want to express. For example, when you talk to a patient about the weather, the patient appears to be listening but in fact, he or she doesn't understand what the word "weather" means. On the other hand, a patient may want to talk about the weather but he or she uses nonsensical speech or a different word unrelated to the word "weather."

Moreover, patients develop apraxia. When this happens, patients have difficulty performing motor functions, despite intact musculoskeletal functioning. If you tell your elderly relative, for example, to unbutton her coat or to comb her hair, she performs the task in an awkward manner despite having no weakness or paralysis of the arms. Agnosia also happens when patients develop inability to recognize familiar objects. If coins, keys, pen, and key chains are placed in their hands, patients cannot recognize them without looking at the objects. Occasionally, they cannot recognize themselves in the mirror. Problems with executive functioning occur when patients have difficulty organizing tasks, things and activities. A well-organized person, for example, becomes disorganized and "messy" in arranging clothes, socks, and underwear. They may be unable to write a check despite having done this activity for many years.

Impairment of abstract thinking eventually occurs. When this happens, patients interpret statements, things and events literally. For example, a patient who is asked to interpret the proverb "don't cry over spilled milk" answers by saying "you just have to wipe it up." When asked to tell the similarity between baseball and basketball, instead of saying "both are sports" they would probably say "both need a ball." Inability to do simple calculation bothers many patients. They used to do subtraction easily but when you ask them to take away 3 from 30, they have difficulty doing so. Attention and concentration are likewise impaired. A female patient, for example, might complain about having difficulty reading a book or newspaper, or struggling to finish the quilt she started a few months ago.

Case scenario

Ms. R's memory worsened gradually. She could not name familiar objects anymore such as chair and watch. She needed help in dressing and taking a bath. Occasionally, she would wet her bed. Her husband hired two caretakers just to help him provide for her basic needs. He was very stressed by Ms. R's accusation that he was laughing at her behind her back. At night, he was bothered that his wife would frequently look at the ceiling and talk to herself incessantly. Her mumblings were mostly incomprehensible. During the day, she would yell and get agitated each time a caretaker would change her clothes. One caretaker suffered a bruise after Ms. R hit her with a tennis racket she grabbed from the wall.

What are the complications to anticipate?

As dementia becomes worse, it develops other symptoms beside forgetfulness. Some patients harbor delusions. As mentioned earlier, delusions are inappropriate ideas or beliefs that are not compatible with the patient's cultural norm. Patients develop inappropriate thoughts that their neighbors are stealing objects and that their relatives are after their money, that people are talking about them or laughing at them. Occasionally, they have thoughts that their spouses are impostors or that their spouses are cheating on them. They experience hallucinations, mostly visual in type. They claim to see relatives who died years ago. Eventually, patients develop behavioral changes such as becoming agitated or aggressive. Some patients spit on or hit their caretakers when being washed and dressed. Others yell the whole day or wander around their house for many hours without getting tired.

What illnesses show dementia?

Alzheimer's disease and vascular dementia are the most common memory disorders but other less common causes include several medical and neurologic conditions such as Parkinson's disease and dementia with lewy bodies.

Alzheimer's Disease

Alzheimer's disease is a type of illness manifested by a gradual deterioration of the memory along with other cognitive, functional, behavioral and emotional impairments. Cognitive changes include apraxia, aphasia, and agnosia, and problems with executive functioning. Once patients develop the cognitive problems, functional impairment ensues. At this time, patients are not able to do their routine activities. Cooking becomes a problem since patients cannot remember the menu and writing a check is a struggle since basic mathematical ability is almost impossible. Behavioral problems such as agitation, wandering, and yelling may occur. At some point, patients undergo emotional changes as manifested by depression, tearfulness, paranoia, anxiety, and even hallucinations.

Dementia affects around 0.5 to 1% of the population and about 5% of people over 65 years old. The most common of all dementias is Alzheimer's disease, comprising about 60% of the demented population. As such, Alzheimer's is a significant cause of morbidity and mortality. The cause of this illness is still unknown. Several risk factors, such as the presence of apolipoprotein E4 and advancing age, have been implicated in its cause. A possible genetic component in its transmission should be considered since mutations in chromosomes 14 and 19 have been associated with familial early onset and familial late onset of this illness, respectively. Moreover, chromosome 21 trisomy is considered as another major risk factor. Neuron loss, plaques, and neurofibrillary tangles, which are anatomic changes found in the brain among Alzheimer's patient, are not diagnostic of the disease because even a healthy elderly person may exhibit these brain changes. Alzheimer's disease is a progressive illness that can result in mortality 8 to 20 years after the initial manifestation or diagnosis of the illness. Mild cognitive disorder is known to precede the illness. Death may be caused by pneumonia due to aspiration. Treatment includes cholinesterase inhibitors, Vitamin E, and orientation aids, among others.

DSM -IV Diagnostic Criteria for Dementia of the Alzheimer's Type

A. The development of multiple cognitive deficits manifested by both
1) memory impairment (impaired ability to learn new information or to recall previously learned information)
2) one (or more) of the following cognitive disturbances:
    a) aphasia (language disturbance)

b) apraxia (impaired ability to carry out motor activities despite intact motor function)

c) agnosia (failure to recognize or identify objects despite intact sensory function)

d) disturbance in executive functioning (i.e. planning, organizing, sequencing, abstracting)

B. The cognitive deficits in Criteria A1 and A2 each cause significant impairment in social or occupational functioning and represent a significant decline from a previous level of functioning.

C. The course is characterized by gradual onset and continuing cognitive decline.

D. The cognitive deficits in Criteria A1 and A2 are not due to any of the following:

1) other central nervous system conditions that cause progressive deficits in memory and cognition (e.g. cerebrovascular disease, Parkinson's disease, Huntington's disease, subdural hematoma, normal-pressure hydrocephalus, brain tumor)

2) systemic conditions that are known to cause dementia (e.g. hypothyroidism, vitamin B12 or folic acid deficiency, niacin deficiency, hypercalcemia, neurosyphylis, HIV infection)

3) substance-induced conditions

E. The deficits do not occur exclusively during the course of a delirium.

F. The disturbance is not better accounted for by another Axis I disorder (e.g. Major Depressive Disorder, Schizophrenia).

Reprinted with permission from the Diagnostic and Statistical Manual of Mental Disorders, Fourth Edition, Text Revision. Copyright 2000. American Psychiatric Association.

Vascular Dementia

Vascular dementia is the second most common type of dementia and is more common among men. It is a type of dementia that is preceded by a stroke or cerebrovascular disease (CVA) caused by blood vessel clogging and bleeding in the brain. The most common cause of vascular dementia is multiple brain infarcts or lesions. The clinical changes found in patients are almost the same as those of Alzheimer's disease such as memory loss, apraxia, functional problems, and emotional symptoms. However, memory loss among vascular dementia patients typically occurs abruptly and progresses in a step-wise fashion. The cognitive deficits are associated with deficits in one part or area of the patient's body, or with multiple lesions in the brain as shown by brain imaging. Medical factors, such as high blood pressure, obesity, high cholesterol (bad cholesterol), heart disease (especially irregular heart rate), diabetes, low oxygen supply due to a chest illness, cigarette smoking and alcohol use increase the chance of patients of developing cerebrovascular disease. Treatment includes a trial of cholinesterase inhibitor, orientation aids, and others.

Other Conditions That Can Manifest As Dementia

Dementia with lewy bodies, traumatic dementia, Pick's disease, Parkinson's disease, alcoholic dementia, metabolic dementia, brain tumor, and delirium are some of the conditions that cause significant memory loss, disorientation, concentration and attention problems, and significant impairment in functioning.

Early intervention

For patients:

- Apply the HEAL technique.

- Accept forgetfulness, impairment in functioning, and other symptoms of dementia, and deal with them.

- Make a will, health care proxy or power of attorney as early as you can while your memory is still intact.

- Make use of memory aids, such as to-do lists, a white board with list of chores, phone and address books, grocery lists, and other kinds of reminders.

- Learn as much as you can about the illness. Visit the library. Contact community organizations and support groups that deal with this type of illness.

- Comply with the medication. Make sure that you take the medication regularly as prescribed by your physician.

- Ask someone to accompany or even drive you when you travel. Have your physician assess you for driving capability.

- Try mental exercise, such as doing crossword puzzles, and reading uplifting books and magazines to stimulate your brain. Don't worry about making mistakes. Just have fun and enjoy.

- Deal with anger and irritability through anger management. Example:
    > You notice that you easily get angry and impatient with your grandchildren. Before saying anything, choose to go to your room and keep your cool.

- For sleep problems, apply sleep hygiene.

- Deal with anxiety through the use of relaxation techniques such as breathing exercises and progressive muscle relaxation.

- Deal with inappropriate thought via thought restructuring. Example:
    > When you become frustrated by the loss of your memory, keep your focus on your hobbies and chores.

- Identify activities that make you feel better. Establish hobbies and other recreational activities such as listening to soothing music, drawing, and baking as a daily routine.

- Recognize and address the triggers of emotional difficulties such as agitation, depression, anger, and anxiety. By recognizing the cause, you may be able to create preventive measures.

- Call a hospital emergency room, crisis line, or mental health services for help. Have yourself assessed by your family physician or a specialist.

- Ask for support and help from the family members. Some relatives are willing to share their time and resources. They can help you in many ways such as buying groceries and arranging your home to meet your needs and keep you safe.

- Organize mental and physical activities into a routine.

- Avoid the use of mood-altering substances such as alcohol and other illicit drugs as a way of dealing with the illness. Using substances only adds to your memory loss.

• Immerse yourself in pleasant and positive thoughts. Negative and self-critical thoughts will make you feel worse.

• Strongly consider going to the hospital when you recognize complications of the illness.

• Renew or strengthen your spirituality. Being connected with the higher power offers hope, inner confidence, guidance, and comfort.

For Caregivers:

• Apply the HELP method.

• Accept forgetfulness, difficulty in functioning, and other symptoms of dementia. Consider them as manifestations of the illness that need to be addressed.

• Recognize and address the triggers of distress, agitation, and other mood problems.
Example:
> You notice that the patient is getting irritable and easily frustrated every morning during bath time. You decide to look at the problem and propose a solution. You notice that the bathroom is not warm enough for the patient's comfort. Moreover, bathroom amenities such as soap and shampoo are not easy to reach. Besides, there are no rails to support the patient in standing up or sitting down. You therefore decide to make changes such as putting up rails, keeping a comfortable bathroom temperature, and making sure that soap and shampoo can easily be grasped.

• Contain inappropriate behavior such as disrobing in public and sexual impropriety. For severe cases, make sure that the patient stays inside the house by installing effective locks. You may also contact the hospital or mental health services for options.

• Monitor the patient for behavioral changes such as pacing back and forth, repetitive movements, and agitation.

• Advice the patient to make a will, power of attorney, and health care proxy while memory is still intact.

- Administer the dementia medication prescribed by the physician (if the patient is unable to) or encourage medication self-management.

- Avoid arguments, confrontations, and criticisms. Help minimize distress in the family.

- Determine medication side effects, such as nausea and vomiting, diarrhea, and weight loss.

- Be alert for signs of threat to self or self-destructive behavior such as giving away possessions, taking a gun out of the cabinet, unprovoked agitation and violence, and unsafe driving. Be alert for any agitated or aggressive behavior as shown by pacing back and forth, easily getting upset for no reason, and becoming verbally abusive.

- Encourage the avoidance of mood-altering substances such as alcohol, and other illicit drugs since using substances only aggravates the situation.

- Check for the early presence of hallucinations and delusions such as talking to oneself and inappropriate fears and beliefs.

- Check for worsening of symptoms, for example, inability to recognize close relatives, disheveled appearance, wandering behavior, and inability to do usual activities such as making the bed or making phone calls.

- Call a hospital emergency room, crisis line, or police officers for help if there is an imminent danger to self or others or inability to take care of oneself.

- Clarify treatment compliance. Ask the patient if he or she has been taking the medications prescribed by the physician.

- Communicate needs, such as housing and personal caretaker, to government agencies.

- Show calendar, familiar pictures and personal mementos to orient patient.

- Encourage socialization and maintenance of usual community activities such as going to church (with supervision if necessary).

- Attend to the patient's personal hygiene, food, health and medical needs.

- Assist in recognizing and addressing problems and issues, for instance anger and agitation, including possible triggers or precipitants.
Example:
> You notice that the patient becomes agitated when a teenage son plays loud rock music. You decide to tell your son to listen to the music in his bedroom.

- Help the patient cope with the hallucinations and delusions through behavioral intervention. Let the patient listen to the radio or be involved in activities when experiencing hallucinations. If the patient becomes suspicious or delusional, offer alternative explanations.

- Allow person to talk and share emotions at a certain time of the day. At this time, focus on patient's concerns and issues. Let the patient talk about frustrations and anger associated with the memory loss. Communicate with the patient through use of simple, understandable words. Be warm, open, and gentle.

- Identify recreational activities and coping strategies that are helpful to the patient. Play soothing music and encourage hobbies previously enjoyed such as quilting or knitting.

- Have the patient evaluated by the family physician or a specialist for the capacity to drive a vehicle. If patient lacks the capacity to drive, offer alternative means of transportation.

- Organize household items for the patients by putting names, signs, or labels on doors, drawers, cabinets, and closets.

- Ensure patient's safety. Make the house safe for daily activities by keeping mechanical tools, sharp objects, cigarettes, medications and poisonous substances away from the patient. Install rails and supports in areas the patient visits frequently such as dining room, the hallway, bedroom, and bathroom. Closely supervise the patient in using the stove or hot water. For wandering patients, make sure that locks (or even alarms) are put in doors and windows so that the patient can't go outside unnoticed.

• Help the patient in various phases of the illness through the application of simple behavioral intervention and coping mechanisms.

• Strongly consider hospitalizing the patient if you observe complications of the illness such as aggression or violence, hallucinations, delusions, and inability to take care of oneself.

Chapter 19

Grief and Bereavement

Case Scenario

Mr. Q, a 65-year-old retired teacher, was apparently doing well until about three weeks ago when his wife of forty years passed away from cancer. He said that their marriage was great and that they had raised five wonderful children, now all married and with children. They struggled financially in the initial years of marriage but by hard work they became prosperous. After their retirement, they traveled to various places in Europe, Asia, the Middle East, and North America. Now he felt very sad that she passed away so soon.

It was difficult for Mr. Q to cope. He would burst into tears at any time of the day. A few days after the burial, he felt very weak. He felt he needed to push himself to go to work, and he could barely concentrate on his tasks. At night, he tossed and turned and hardly slept. Occasionally, he would experience hearing "the voice" of his wife calling his name. Six to seven weeks after her death, Mr. Q gradually felt better. He said that he was not crying as much. His strength was almost returning to normal. He eventually returned to work in a better emotional state.

How is the illness manifested?

Grief and bereavement is a condition or state which follows the loss of a loved one. After the death of a loved one, patients develop a range of emotional difficulties. A state of denial occurs, a period when people have difficulty accepting the loss. Some patients feel angry at the loss and its associated consequences, such as the loss of a vital source of support, diminished comfort and security, and loss of romantic relationship. After the loss, a period of instability usually sets in among family members. This period of abrupt change and instability can cause significant emotional suffering. Some patients develop depression, irritability, and anxiety about the future. As time passes, patients become more accepting of the loss and decide to move on with their lives.

Case scenario

Four months after the death of his wife, Mr. Q remained depressed and tearful and his energy level was very low. In fact, every morning after waking up, he preferred to simply lie down on the couch. He would not do anything, not even cook his food or do the laundry. He lost much weight since he had not eaten well since his wife's death. His sleep had also been terrible.

A month later, he further deteriorated. He felt worthless, "like a piece of junk." He thought that nobody could help him. Gradually, he began to believe that he was better off dead. He felt so hopeless that he couldn't see any "light at the end of the tunnel." He thought of joining his wife in heaven. He became so preoccupied with her that he made plans to hurt himself.

What are the complications to anticipate?

Clinical depression may set in if the emotional difficulties are prolonged and not addressed by mental health professionals. The appearance of neurovegetative signs and symptoms, such as lack of sleep, poor energy, inability to concentrate, loss of libido, and lack of appetite, is common. Patients develop feelings of hopelessness, worthlessness, and helplessness. Some may even experience thoughts of deaths and suicidal behavior. Others develop prolonged and intense anxiety symptoms such as panic attacks, agitation, feeling edgy and tense, and palpitations. Those patients who desire relief from their distress become involved in heavy alcohol and drug use.

Some patients who have lost their loved one through violent death, accident or suicide, experience symptoms consistent with posttraumatic stress disorder, such as nightmares and clear and graphic recollection of the event. Furthermore, a protracted course of bereavement results in medical complications such as gradual deterioration of health, increased risk to develop heart disease, vague bodily symptoms, and occasionally death due to medical problems (especially for elderly), suicide, or accidents.

What illnesses may manifest the signs and symptoms of grief and bereavement?

Conditions that may mimic grief and bereavement include major depressive disorder, adjustment disorder, and anxiety disorders.

Grief and Bereavement

Grief and bereavement is a normal process that occurs after the death of a loved one. Emotional instability in the form of sadness, tearfulness, inability to sleep and eat, and feelings of anger and guilt, develops. In general, grief lasts for about one to two months but for some people, it may last for about a year. Cultural context should also be taken into account in understanding the grieving process. Although some individuals need counseling to help them cope with the loss, most people move on with their normal lives after a few months without professional help.

Major Depressive Disorder

Occasionally, the normal grieving process turns into a worse condition and becomes "pathological." In an abnormal state, the grieving process becomes prolonged, impairing the health and functioning of the individual, and becoming associated with prolonged neurovegetative signs and symptoms such as sleep, appetite, and energy impairment. Individuals may later develop the psychological symptoms of hopelessness, worthlessness, and even thoughts of death. This abnormal state can now be considered as more than just simple grief and may meet clinical depression criteria. When this is the case, the patient is treated with medications and psychotherapy.

Adjustment Disorder

After the death of a loved one, emotional difficulties such as anger, sadness, anxiety, or behavioral changes ensue resulting in impairment in functioning or excessive distress. These difficulties however should be resolved within three months after the loss. If symptoms persist beyond three months, another psychiatric disorder may have developed. (Please see the adjustment disorder discussion in previous chapters.)

Grief and Bereavement

Anxiety Disorder

Consider the presence of an anxiety disorder when the anxiety symptoms such as excessive worrying, lack of sleep and concentration, and feelings of restlessness become overwhelming and cause significant dysfunction and distress. When avoidance, nightmares, and graphic recollection of sudden and violent death occur, posttraumatic stress disorder is mostly likely present. Medications and psychotherapy may be tried for both conditions. (Please see anxiety disorder and posttraumatic stress disorder discussion in previous chapters.)

Early intervention

For Patients:

- Apply the HEAL technique.

- Accept tearfulness, irritability, anxiety, anger, and other symptoms as part of grieving.

- Review helpful coping strategies in the past that can be used at present.
Example:
> If you have felt better talking with friends about your problems in the past, then talk to friends about your concerns now.

- Recognize changes in emotion and behavior when you are reminded of a deceased loved one.

- Encourage a gathering of family members.

- Have plenty of rest, nutritious food, and sleep.

- Mourn the loss at a specified time each day. Scheduling your mourning gives you more control of your emotions and ultimately your life. You can, however, decide to be more flexible, if need be.
Example:
> You may decide to mourn the loss of your loved one everyday for one hour at around 8 PM.

- Say goodbye through appropriate gestures, such as writing a goodbye letter, expressing your emotions in a journal, visiting the cemetery, and praying for the deceased.

- Read the literature such as books, magazines, newspapers, and newsletters about grief and how to cope with it.

- Comply with the medication. Make sure that you take the medication regularly as prescribed by your physician.

- Deal with anger and irritability through anger management.
Example:
> You feel angry for the loss of your loved one. You decide to release your anger by writing your anger in a journal and by punching your pillow.

- For sleep problems, apply sleep hygiene.

- Deal with anxiety through the use of relaxation techniques such as breathing exercises and progressive muscle relaxation.

- Deal with depression by focusing on pleasant thoughts such as golden moments together with your loved one.

- Deal with inappropriate thought by thought restructuring.
Example:
> Your mind is too preoccupied with the manner in which your loved one died. When this happens, anger and depression set in. Decide to change your mindset by focusing on the pleasant moments together with your deceased loved one.

- Identify activities that make you feel better. If regular walks in the morning perks you up, then establish this routine.

- Recognize and address triggers of emotional difficulties which complicate your current grief. By recognizing the cause, you may be able to create preventive measures. If a conflict with a co-worker precipitates your relapse, try to improve your work relationship through improved communication.

- Cope with suicidal thoughts through diversion: physical diversion involves activities such as recreational activities, going out, and exercise; social diversion includes visiting your friends and relatives; and mental diversion consists of mental activities such as thought replacement. Telling your relative and therapist about thoughts of self-harm is beneficial in getting immediate help.

• Call a hospital emergency room, crisis line, or mental health services for help.

• Ask for support from family members. Some relatives are willing to share their time and resources in helping you manage your concerns.

• Delay making major decisions while still in distress. The majority of people can't make rational choices when the mind is impaired by illness.

• Organize daily activities and routine.

• Avoid putting yourself down. Don't blame yourself for the death of your loved one.

• Avoid the use of mood-altering substances such as alcohol and other illicit drugs as a way of dealing with the loss. Using substances only adds to the problem.

• Immerse yourself in pleasant and positive thoughts. Negative and self-critical thoughts will make you feel worse.

• Strongly consider going to the hospital when complications of the illness arise.

• Renew or strengthen your spirituality. Being connected with the higher power offers hope, inner confidence, guidance, and comfort.

For Caregivers:

• Apply the HELP method.

• Accept depression, tearfulness, anxiety, anger, irritability, and other symptoms of grief and then deal with them.

- Assist in getting a mental health assessment by a professional and support services. Offer to look for available mental health resources in the community and make the initial phone calls to set up an appointment.

- Help the patient organize personal undertakings such as paying bills, and making an appointment with health care professionals.

- Allow the patient to talk about the details of the death of a loved one and its associated emotions, and memories of the deceased (use of mementos/photo album, and so on). Help the patient obtain more information about the cause of death. Let him or her know that expressing a variety of emotions is okay.

- Provide comfort and help the patient feel safe and secure.

- Advise patient not to put blame on self.

- Encourage the patient to mourn daily at a particular time.

- Encourage plenty of rest, nutritious food, and sleep.

- Allow the person to talk and share emotions at a certain time of the day. At this time, focus on the patient's concerns and issues.

- Help administer the medication prescribed by the physician (if the patient is unable to) or encourage medication self-management.

- Clarify safety by asking about the presence of suicidal or homicidal thoughts. Asking this question will not encourage patients to hurt themselves or others.

- Be alert for signs of threat to self or self-destructive behavior such as superficial cuts in the wrist, empty bottles next to the bed, goodbye letters, giving away possessions, or taking a gun out of the cabinet. Be alert for any agitated or aggressive behavior as shown by pacing back and forth, easily getting upset for no reason, and becoming verbally abusive.

- Encourage the avoidance of mood-altering substances such as alcohol and other illicit drugs as a way of coping with the problem. Remind the patient that using substances only aggravates the situation.

Grief and Bereavement

- Call a hospital emergency room, crisis line, or police officers for help if there is an imminent danger to self or others.

- Clarify treatment compliance. Ask the patient if he/she has been taking the medications prescribed by the physician.

- Encourage patient to read the literature and to attend seminars or support groups on grief.

- Ask for support from family members. Help in conveying messages to friends and relatives. Some patients prefer to be in the company of caring people during these difficult times.

- Advise the patient to delay making major decisions while in distress. Make the patient realize that emotional difficulties can impair judgment and affect the decision-making process.

- Reinforce coping skills and positive messages. Appreciate patients' efforts to help themselves, such as through improved nutrition and sleep, participation in activities, and writing journals.

- Build the patient's hopes. Share your own experiences about how you successfully dealt with emotional difficulties in the past. Remind the patient that current difficulties are just temporary. If the patient has an appointment with a health care professional, reassure him/her that help is coming soon.

- Help the patient organize a daily routine. Assist patients who lack the motivation and energy to establish structure by writing to-do lists and making appointments.

- Avoid arguments, confrontations, and criticisms. This is not the best time to engage in fruitless communication.

- Help the patient in applying for sick or emergency leave.

- Strongly consider hospitalizing the patient if you observe complications of the illness.

Chapter 20

Commonly Asked Questions and Related Issues

What are the indications for hospitalization?

Hospitalization is indicated for patients who suffer from moderate to severe mental illness, especially if associated with a significant lack of understanding about the illness, substantial suicidal or homicidal risk, and considerable deterioration in functioning. This treatment intervention should also be considered in other situations, such as the need to observe the patient's clinical status and to monitor and treat side effects. Initial administration of medication, lack of support from family members, complicated psychiatric condition, unpredictable behavioral problems, unresponsiveness and noncompliance to outpatient treatment, and respite from a stressful situation are also acceptable indications for hospitalization.

What are the indications for outpatient clinic?

Outpatient treatment is indicated for patients with good family support, adequate coping mechanisms, and mild to moderate severity of the illness. Moreover, lack of stressors in the home environment, adequate understanding about the illness, and intact ability to care for oneself are good reasons to treat the individual as outpatient.

What is civil commitment or involuntary hospitalization? When can this be applied?

Civil commitment is another term for involuntary hospitalization. It has two components: first, the presence of mental illness, and second, a threat to self or others. Some jurisdictions accept the inability to care for oneself as the second component. Involuntary hospitalization can be applied only if the patient's mental illness is associated with a significant degree of threat to oneself or others. Most jurisdictions require that there should be convincing proof of the threat or that an imminent threat exists. Since the liberty of the patient is at stake, the mere thought or verbalization of a threat does not usually qualify. Likewise, a threat to self or others, without associated mental illness, is not an indication for involuntary hospitalization.

A question can be raised as to whether keeping certified psychiatric patients in jail for a long period of time while awaiting bed availability in the hospital is justified, especially if these patients have no criminal charges. As a rule, psychiatric patients who are certified or committed and under police custody due to significant threat to self or others should be brought to the hospital. It is the duty of the physician to place the certified patient in a secure place. Occasionally however, some certified patients end up in jail for several hours, at times more than 24 hours, after being turned down for admission by a psychiatric institution due to lack of bed availability, inadequate observation/holding areas, or lack of staff.

It is unethical and malpractice to put a mentally ill patient in jail while awaiting hospital bed availability. A jail should never be used as a substitute or replacement when observation rooms in the emergency area, adequate staffing, and hospital beds are lacking. A jail cannot provide the comfort and safety that mentally ill patients need at this difficult time. Moreover, the patient may suffer significantly while under the care of staffs with no medical or adequate mental health training. For instance, one psychotic patient committed suicide while being "closely" watched by a police officer. Furthermore, being incarcerated may seriously increase the stigma commonly associated with mental illness.

A health care professional or institution that regularly or even occasionally uses jail as a treatment option or "holding area" for various reasons, such as waiting for bed availability, is open to unlimited liability. The institution or healthcare professional may be sued for false or forced imprisonment, lack of assessment, and inadequate treatment intervention. The health care professional may be subject to an ethical inquiry and a license review by the medical board for providing inappropriate intervention for a patient.

What is informed consent?

Informed consent is a doctrine that allows patients to exercise free will in determining the best treatment option for their medical condition. This doctrine has three components. According to Dr. Simon (2001), patients should have the capacity to make a decision, that adequate information is given to them, and that they should give their consent or permission voluntarily, without any form of force or coercion from anyone, especially from the health care professional. In the absence of any of these components, informed consent is not possible. A patient who lacks decisional capacity, for instance, cannot give an informed consent even if this patient receives a substantial amount of information and wants to give consent voluntarily.

A patient manifests decisional capacity if he or she has an adequate understanding of the issues and can appreciate the available options. The patient must be able to make a choice and should have the capability to express that choice. For example, a depressed lawyer visits a renowned psychiatrist. After an hour of evaluation, the physician gives the patient drug treatment options, such as the use of Venlafaxine, Paroxetine, and Mirtazapine and describes the advantages and disadvantages of each drug. The lawyer meticulously weighs the pros and cons of each option. He decides to use Venlafaxine due to its low potential to interact with his other medications and its high rate of remission. He then conveys his choice to his psychiatrist.

A health care professional is expected to provide adequate information to patients. Be aware that just having the patient sign a consent form without giving information is not informed consent. How much information is adequate remains a matter of controversy. It is, however, reasonable for the physician to explain the medical findings, the psychiatric diagnosis, treatment options and their associated advantages and disadvantages, the short-term and long-term side effects of the procedure or medication, and the possible outcome with or without the use of the treatment recommendations. For example, a female celebrity with a severe form of psychotic disorder is not responding to any medication. Her psychiatrist discusses the possible role of electroconvulsive therapy for this type of condition. The physician further explains why the procedure is necessary and describes its risks and benefits.

The patient's permission should be free from intimidation and unnecessary influence. Even small hints of blackmail should be avoided. An elderly female patient in a nursing home, for instance, should not be coerced to take medication by implying that her monthly check will be withheld if she refuses to take the pill.

Dr. Simon lists four exceptions to informed consent: first, emergency situations such as an imminent threat to oneself or others; secondly, lack of decisional capacity or incompetence; thirdly, therapeutic privilege – a concept that allows clinicians not to divulge information to the patient if, in their judgment, the new information would be deleterious to the health of the patient; and lastly, waiver. In the latter's case, the patient makes a competent decision not to obtain any information about the treatment or procedure at issue.

What is the responsibility of the physician before dispensing medication?

The physician has the responsibility to explain adequately the following information: 1) the nature and possible causes of the mental condition necessitating medication; 2) the medication and its mechanism of action, frequency of intake, and the time when it begins to work; 3) the side effect profile of the drug; 4) the risks and benefits involved in the use of the specific medication; 5) alternative treatment interventions and their risks and benefits; and 6) the prognosis (or possible outcome) with or without treatment intervention. In addition, the clinician should emphasize treatment compliance. Dispensing prescription, without educating the patient adequately, frequently results in noncompliance.

What are the common reasons for failure of drug treatment?

There are many reasons why mentally ill patients do not respond well to drug treatment. 1) The patient may not be properly assessed by the physician resulting in wrong diagnosis and inadequate appreciation of the ongoing issues. 2) The patient may not be taking the correct medication for the illness. Instead of taking antidepressants for clinical depression, for instance, the patient is taking benzodiazepines, an anti-anxiety medication. 3) The patient may not be taking the correct dose of the medication. For example, a 40-year-old depressed patient is started on a small dose of SSRIs such as 10 mg/day rather than the usual starting dose of 20 mg/day.

4) The patient may not be taking the medication regularly. Most psychotropic medications do not work properly if not taken daily. Antidepressant medications, for instance, do not work if given or taken on an as-needed basis. Medications should maintain an adequate level in the body in order to work properly. 5) The patient may require a combination of medications rather than just one medication. For example, a psychotic patient who feels depressed requires an antipsychotic medication along with an antidepressant.

6) The patient may have more than one mental disorder. For instance, a patient suffering from obsessive-compulsive disorder may also be suffering from generalized anxiety disorder, and may require a drug treatment for both disorders. 7) It is also likely that the mentally ill patient is involved in the heavy use of alcohol or illicit drugs. This condition further complicates

the clinical picture and response to drug treatment. 8) The patient may be suffering from a personality disorder, a condition that is in general difficult to treat, along with a psychiatric disorder. 9) The patient may have a serious medical problem that contributes to the emotional problem. For instance, an anxious patient with hyperthyroidism will not respond to anti-anxiety medication unless the medical condition is treated. And 10) the patient may be affected by a lot of stressors, such as marital and financial problems. In order to treat the condition successfully, these issues should be addressed. No amount of medication can cure a failing marriage.

What are the options for patients not responding properly to a specific type of medication?

For patients who do not respond to a particular type of medication, the reasons for drug failure (as stated above) should first be adequately addressed by the physician. Several options can still be tried. First, the dose of the medication can be increased. For example, a patient has taken 30 mg of paroxetine per day for almost three months with minimal response. The dose may then be increased to 40 mg per day. Secondly, another medication can be added to augment the effect of the current medication or to treat another symptom. If, for example, the patient who takes paroxetine 40 mg per day still does not respond, the physician may try adding lithium carbonate. A trazodone may be added to paroxetine to address insomnia. Thirdly, the current medication can be switched to another medication that belongs to a different class. For example, paroxetine is switched to venlafaxine if no adequate response is observed after sufficient trial.

What are some of the emergency or crisis situations?

The common crisis or emergency situations include suicidal or homicidal risk, behavioral changes including aggression, significant deterioration in functioning, severe form of the mental illness such as psychosis, drug and alcohol-related problems such as intoxication, withdrawal signs and symptoms, and delirium, toxicity from a medication such as lithium, significant side effects from the medication such as acute dystonia from neuroleptics, drug interactions, and serious family and marital conflict.

What is confidentiality?

Confidentiality is the responsibility and obligation of the clinician to keep private all information disclosed by the patient. Confidentiality is important in maintaining and improving the therapeutic environment since it allows the patient to express emotional and physical distress without fear of being the subject of public scrutiny. Free flow of information in a treatment setting is critical in providing the health care professional with ample opportunity to make an appropriate assessment and treatment recommendations.

Information can only be released to a third party with the patient's written permission or consent. Without appropriate consent, clinicians open themselves to malpractice liability. Verbal consent is not adequate to safeguard privacy and will not protect the clinician from a potential lawsuit. Written consent is the most valid and acceptable approach in our litigious culture.

There are, however, several exceptions to confidentiality. They include emergency situations such as a substantial threat to self or others, elder or child abuse, court-ordered evaluations, and infectious disease such as tuberculosis. Always be mindful of the acceptable exceptions in your jurisdiction.

What is privilege?

Privilege or testimonial privilege is the right of the patient to prevent one's physician to disclose any clinical information in court. This concept is important in protecting the doctor-patient relationship from court intrusion. Exceptions to privilege include court-ordered evaluations and reports, and civil and criminal proceedings, among others.

Does the patient have the right to refuse treatment?

A patient has the right to refuse treatment if there is no emergency and if one's decision-making capacity is intact. In situations where there is serious mental illness associated with an imminent danger to self or others and lack of decisional capacity, medication may be administered temporarily. But once the crisis is over and the patient regains capacity to make a decision, informed consent should be given. A patient may then refuse the treatment again.

If the patient has a "permanent" decisional incapacity due to an illness such as severe mental retardation or dementia, a substitute decision maker is necessary. In general, close relatives have a role to play in giving consent. Depending upon the jurisdiction, a guardian may be appointed by the court if a patient is found to be incompetent. The court also determines the need for treatment, and orders the necessary intervention.

How can suicidal or homicidal ideation be assessed and what can you do about it?

Anyone who harbors suicidal or homicidal ideation should be taken seriously and should be asked questions to explore its severity and extent. Determine the frequency of occurrence and the presence of real intent to harm self or others. Ask about any specific plan. Is the person contemplating on hanging oneself, overdosing, or using a gun? Determine the specifics of the plan such as date and place. For example, a patient tells you that his suicidal thoughts have become intense during the past three weeks. Now, he begins to contemplate ending his life by cutting his wrist with a knife while everyone is asleep. Those patients who do not admit having thoughts of self-harm or harming others should be observed closely for any signs of destructive or potentially unsafe gestures such as buying a rope, taking a loaded gun from the cabinet, inflicting superficial lacerations on the wrist, and having empty medication bottles in the bedroom.

Once you determine a potential risk, you should get help as soon as you can. Call the nearest mental health center, crisis center, or hospital. Contact 1-800 hotlines for advice. Meanwhile, keep potential weapons such as knives, blades, medications, guns, and rope away from the patient. Place them in a locked cabinet. Also, observe the patient closely and ascertain his or her safety. Patient who needs help should be taken to the hospital emergency room for evaluation and treatment. However, if a patient becomes an imminent danger to self or others and does not wish to get treatment or be hospitalized, then you may need to call the crisis center or law enforcement agency immediately.

Appendix

Resources for Patients and Caregivers

National Alliance for the Mentally Ill
Colonial Place Three
2107 Wilson Blvd., Suite 300
Arlington, VA 22201-3042
USA
Help Line: 800-950-NAMI (6264)
Main Office: 703-524-7600
Fax: 703 524-9094
Web: www.nami.org

National Mental Health Association
1021 Prince Street
Alexandria, VA 22314-2971
USA
Phone: 800-969-NMHA (6642) or 703-684-7722
Fax: 703-684-5968
Web: www.nmha.org

The World Federation for Mental Health
1021 Prince Street
Alexandria, VA 22314-2971
USA
Fax: 703-519-7648
Web: www.wfmh.com

Canadian Mental Health Association
CMHA National Office
2160 Yonge Street, 3rd Floor
Toronto, ON M4S2Z3
Canada
Phone: 416-484-7750
Fax: 416-484-4617
E-mail: national@cmha.ca
Web: www.cmha.ca

Mood Disorders Association of Manitoba
4-1000 Notre Dame
Winnipeg, Manitoba R3E0N3
Canada
Phone: 800-263-1460 or 204-786-0987
Fax: 204-786-1906
Web: www.depression.mb.ca

National Network for Mental Health
55 King Street, Suite 303
St. Catharine's, ON L2R3H5
Canada
Phone: 888-406-4663 or 905-682-2423
Fax: 905-682-7469
E-mail: member@nnmh.ca
Web: www.nnmh.ca

Alzheimer's Society of Canada
20 Eglinton Ave. W., Suite 1200
Toronto, ON M4R1K8
Canada
Phone: 800-616-8816 or 416-488-8772
Fax: 416-488-3778
E-mail: info@alzheimer.ca
Web: www.alzheimer.ca

Canadian Psychiatric Association
260-441 Maclaren St.
Ottawa, ON K2P2H3
Canada
Phone: 613-234-2815
Fax: 613-234-9857
E-mail: cpa@cpa-apc.org
Web: www.cpa-apc.org

Schizophrenia Society of Canada
75 The Donway west, Suite 814
Don Mills, ON M3C2E9
Phone: 888-SSC-HOPE (772-4673)
E-mail: info@schizophrenia.ca
Phone: 416-445-8204
Web: www.schizophrenia.ca

World Psychiatric Association
International Center for Mental Health
Mount Sinai School of Medicine of New York University
5th Ave and 100 St. PO Box 1093
New York, NY 10029-6574
USA
Web: www.wpanet.org

International Stress Management Association
PO Box 348
Waltham Cross EN88ZL
England
Phone: +44 (0) 7000 780430
Fax: +44 (0) 1992 426673
Web: www.isma.org.uk

Centre for Addiction and Mental health
33 Russell St.
Toronto, ON M5S2S1
Canada
Phone: 800-463-6273 or 416-535-8501 ext. 6111
Web: www.camh.net

Canadian Centre on Substance Abuse
75 Albert St., Suite 300
Ottawa, ON K1P5E7
Canada
Phone: 613-235-4048
Fax: 613-235-8101
Web: www.ccsa.ca

Health Canada
Mental Health Promotion Unit
Jeanne Mance Bldg., 7th floor
Tunney's Pasture
Address locator #1907-C1
Ottawa, ON K1A1B4
Canada
Phone: 613-957-2991
Fax: 613-946-3595
E-mail: mhp@www.hc-sc.gc.ca
Web: www.hc-sc.gc.ca

Al-Anon Family group Headquarters, Inc.
1600 Corporate Landing Parkway
Virginia Beach, VA 23454-5617
USA
Phone: 757-563-1600
Fax: 757-563-1655
E-mail: wso@al-anon.org
Web: www.al-anon.alateen.org

Alzheimer's Association
919 N. Michigan Ave., Suite 1100
Chicago, IL 60611-1676
USA
Phone: 800-272-3900 or 312-335-8700
Fax: 312-335-1110
E-mail: info@alz.org
Web: www.alz.org

American Association of Retired Persons
601 E Street NW
Washington, DC 20049
USA
Phone: 800-424-3410
E-mail: member@aarp.org
Web: www.aarp.org

American Association of Suicidology
4201 Connecticut Ave. NW Suite 408
Washington, DC 20008
USA
Phone: 202-237-2280
Fax: 202-237-2282
E-mail: ajkulp@suicidology.org
Web: www.suicidology.org

Depression and related Affective Disorders Association
Meyer 3-181
600 North Wolfe St.
Baltimore, MD 21287-7381
USA
Phone: 202-955-5800 or 410-955-4647
E-mail: drada@jhmi.edu
Web: www.med.jhu.edu

Institute for Mental Health Initiatives
2175 K St. NW, Suite 700
Washington, DC 20037
USA
Phone: 202-467-2285
Fax: 202-467-2289
E-mail: imhi-info@gwumc.edu
Web: www.gwumc.edu/sphhs/imhi/

Mood Disorders Support Group of New York City
PO Box 30377
New York, NY 10011
USA
Phone: 212-533-6374
Fax: 212-675-0218
E-mail: info@mdsg.org
Web: www.mdsg.org

Narcotics Anonymous
World Service Office in LA
PO Box 9999
Van Nuys, CA 91409
USA
Phone: 818-773-9999
Fax: 818-700-0700
E-mail: fsmail@na.org
Web: www.na.org

National Association for the Dually Diagnosed
132 Fair St.
Kingston, NY 12401-4802
USA
Phone: 800-331-5362 or 845-331-4336
Fax: 845-331-4569
E-mail: thenadd@aol.com
Web: www.thenadd.org

National Association of Anorexia Nervosa and Associated Disorders
PO Box 7
Highland Park, IL 60035
USA
Phone: 847-831-3438(hotline) or 847-831-3438

Fax: 847-433-4632
E-mail: anad20@aol.com
Web: www.anad.org

National Clearinghouse for Alcohol and Drug Information
PO Box 2345
Rockville, MD 20847-2345
USA
Phone: 800-729-6686
E-mail: webmaster@health.org
Web: www.health.org

Alcoholics Anonymous
General Service Office/Grand Central Station
PO Box 459
New York, NY 10163
USA
Phone: 212-870-3400
Fax: 212-870-3003
Web: www.alcoholics-anonymous.org

Marijuana Anonymous
PO Box 2912
Van Nuys, CA 91404
USA
Phone: 800-766-6779
E-mail: office@marijuana-anonymous.org
Web: www.marijuana-anonymous.org

Families Anonymous
PO Box 3475
Culver City, CA 90231-3475
USA
Phone: 8000-736-9805
Fax: 310-815-9682
E-mail: famanon@FamiliesAnonymous.org
Web: www.familiesanonymous.org

National Depressive and Manic-Depressive Association
730 N Franklin St. Suite 501
Chicago, IL 60610-7204
USA
Phone: 800-826-3632 or 312-642-0049

Fax: 312-642-7243
Web: www.nmda.org

National Institute of Mental Health
6001 Executive Blvd., Rm 8184, MSC 9663
Bethesda, MD 20892-9663
USA
Phone: 301-443-4513
Fax: 301-443-4279
E-mail: nimhinfo@nih.gov
Web: www.nimh.nih.gov

Obsessive Compulsive Foundation
337 Notch Hill Road
North Branford, CT 06471
USA
Phone: 203-315-2190
Fax: 203-315-2196
E-mail: info@ocfoundation.org
Web: www.ocfoundation.org

America Foundation for Suicide Prevention
120 Wall St., 22nd floor
New York, NY 10005
USA
Phone: 888-333-AFSP or 212-363-3500
Fax: 212-363-6237
E-mail: inquiry@afsp.org
Web: www.afsp.org

Federation of families for Children's Mental Health
1101 King St., Suite 420
Alexandria, VA 22314
USA
Phone: 703-684-7710
Fax: 703-836-1040
E-mail: ffcmh@ffcmh.org
Web: www.ffcmh.org

The National Information Center for Children and Youth with Disabilities
PO Box 1492
Washington, DC 20013-1492

USA
Phone: 800-695-0285 or 202-884-8200
Fax: 202-884-8441
E-mail: nichcy@aed.org
Web: www.nichcy.org

Anxiety Disorders Association of America
11900 Parklawn Dr., Suite 100
Rockville, MD 20852
USA
Phone: 301-231-9350
Web: www.adaa.org

The National Eating Disorders Association
603 Stewart St., Suite 803
Seattle, WA 98101
USA
Phone: 800-931-2237 or 206-382-3587
Fax: 206-829-8501
E-mail: info@edap.org
Web: www.nationaleatingdisorders.org

The National Eating Disorder Information Center
CW 1-211, 200 Elizabeth St.
Toronto, ON M5G2C4
Canada
Phone: 866-633-4220 or 416-340-4156
E-mail: nedic@uhn.on.ca
Web: www.nedic.ca

Bulimia Anorexia Nervosa Association
300 Cabana Road East
Windsor, ON N9G1A3
Canada
Phone: 519-969-2112
Fax: 519-969-0227
E-mail: info@bana.ca
Web: www.bana.ca

National Family Caregivers Association
10400 Connecticut Ave., #500
Kensington, MD 20895-3944
USA

Resources for Patients and Caregivers

Phone: 800-896-3650
Fax: 301-942-2302
E-mail: info@nfcacares.org
Web: www.nfcacares.org

The Center for Family Caregivers
PO Box 224
Park ridge, IL 60068
USA
Phone: 847-823-0639
E-mail: denise@familycaregivers.org
Web: www.familycaregivers.org

Caregiver's Army
PO Box 64
Berlin Center, OH 44401
USA
E-mail: carladydove1@juno.com
Web: www.caregiversarmy.com

Family Caregiver Alliance
690 Market St., Suite 600
San Francisco, CA 94104
USA
Phone: 415-434-3388
Fax: 415-434-3508
E-mail: info@caregiver.org
Web: www.caregiver.org

Caregiver Network Inc.
561 Avenue Road, Suite 206
Toronto, ON M4V2J8
Canada
Phone: 416-323-1090
Fax: 416-966-2341
E-mail: karenh@caregiver.on.ca
Web: www.caregiver.on.ca

Caregivers.com
17 Applegate Ct
Madison, WI 53713
USA
Phone: 608-256-0488

E-mail: support@bettergiving.com
Web: www.caregivers.com

Well Spouse foundation
Box 30093
Elkins Park, PA 19027
USA
Phone: 800-838-0879
E-mail: info@wellspouse.org
Web: www.wellspouse.org

The Compassionate Friends, Inc.
PO Box 3696
Oak Brook, IL 60522-3696
USA
Phone: 877-969-0010 or 630-990-0010
Fax: 630-990-0246
E-mail: nationaloffice@compassionatefriends.org
Web: www.compassionatefriends.org

The National Council on the Aging
409 Third St. SW, Suite 200
Washington, DC 20024
USA
Phone: 202-479-1200
Fax: 202-479-0735
E-mail: info@ncoa.org
Web: www.ncoa.org

References and Recommended Readings

American Psychiatric Association. Practice Guidelines. Washington, D.C.: APA; 1996

American Psychiatric Association. Practice Guidelines for the Treatment of Patients with Alzheimer's disease and other Dementias of Late Life. Washington, D.C.: APA; 1997.

American Psychiatric Association. Practice Guidelines for the Treatment of Patients with Schizophrenia. Washington, D.C.: APA; 1996.

American Psychiatric Association. Diagnostic and Statistical Manual of Mental Disorders, 4th ed., Text Revision. Washington D.C.: American Psychiatric Association; 2000.

Appelbaum PS, Gutheil TG. Clinical Handbook of Psychiatry and the Law. 2nd ed. Maryland: Williams and Wilkins; 1991.

Beck AT, Rush AJ, Shaw BF, Emery G. Cognitive Therapy of Depression. New York: Guilford Press; 1979.

Bower SA, Bower GH. Asserting Yourself. 2nd ed. Reading, MA: Addison-Wesley; 1991.

Burns DD. The Feeling Good Handbook. New York: Plume; 1989.

Clark DM, Fairburn CG, editors. Science and Practice of Cognitive Behaviour Therapy. New York: Oxford University Press; 1997.

Ectasia. Dorland's illustrated medical dictionary. 28th ed. Philadelphia: Saunders; 1994.

Fanning F, McKay M, editors. Family Guide to Emotional Wellness. Oakland, CA: New Harbinger; 2000.

Flaherty JA, Davis JM, Janicak PG. Psychiatry Diagnosis and Therapy. 2nd ed. Norwalk, CT: Appleton & Lange; 1993.

Frances A, Ross R. DSM IV Case Studies: A Clinical Guide to Differential Diagnosis. Washington, D.C.: American Psychiatric Press; 1996.

First MB, Frances A, Pincus HA. DSM IV Handbook of Differential Diagnosis. Washington, D.C.: American Psychiatric Press; 1995.

Kaplan HI, Sadock BJ. Synopsis of Psychiatry. 8th ed. Maryland: Williams and Wilkins; 1998.

Kaplan HI, Sadock BJ, editors. Comprehensive Textbook of Psychiatry. 6th ed. Maryland: Williams and Wilkins; 1995.

McCann-Beranger J. A Caregiver's Guide for Alzheimer Disease and Other Dementias. Charlottetown, PEI: Alzheimer Society; 2000.

Novales PN, Rojcewicz SJ, Peeles R. Clinical Manual of Supportive Psychotherapy. Washington D.C.: American Psychiatric Press; 1993.

Pollack MH, Otto MW, Rosenbaum JF, editors. Challenges in Clinical Practice. New York: Guilford Press; 1996.

Sadavoy J, Lazarus LW, Jarvik LF, Grossberg GT, editors. Comprehensive Review of Geriatric Psychiatry. 2nd ed. Washington D.C.: American Psychiatric Press; 1996.

Schuckit MA. Drug and Alcohol Abuse. 3rd ed. New York: Plenum Publishing; 1989.

Sharfstein SS, Webb WL, Stoline AM. Economics of Psychiatry. In: Kaplan HI, Sadock BJ, editors. Comprehensive Textbook of Psychiatry. 6th ed. Maryland: Williams and Wilkins; 1995: 2677-2689.

Simon RI. Concise Guide to Psychiatry and Law for Clinicians. 3rd ed. Washington, D.C.: American Psychiatric Press; 2001.

Stern TA, Herman JB, Slavin PL, editors. The MGH Guide to Psychiatry in Primary Care. New York: Mc-Graw Hill; 1998.

Rayel MG. Successful Preparation for the Psychiatry Oral Exam: How to Effectively Organize Your Interview, Oral Presentation, and Video Exam. Newfoundland: Soar Dime; 2001.

Wolpe J. The Practice of Behavior Therapy. 2nd ed. New York: Pergamon Press; 1973.

Index

A

ABCs, first aid 22-27
Active listening 41
Activity scheduling 44
Actual exposure 30, 31, 32, 33
Acute stress disorder 96
Address the issues 20
Adjustment disorder 54, 106, 154
After trauma, early intervention for patients 96 for caregivers 99
Agnosia 143, 144
Agoraphobia 79
Alcohol abuse 122
    Complications 123
    Early intervention for patients 128 for caregivers 130
Alcohol dependence 122
    Complications 123
    Early intervention for patients 128 for caregivers 130
Alternative behavior 40
Alzheimer's disease 144
    Risk factors 144
Amphetamines 124
Anger management 39-41, 55, 64, 97, 117, 129, 138, 147, 156
Anorexia nervosa 135
    Causes 135
    Diagnostic criteria 135-136
Anticipate complications 8
Anxiety disorder 155
    Changes 103
    Complications 103
    Early intervention for patients 106 for caregivers
Anxiety disorder, medical condition 105

Aphasia 143, 144
Apraxia 143, 144
Assessment, suicidal or homical ideation 165
Assertiveness technique 38
Auditory hallucination 51, 111
Availability 24

B

Binge eating 134
Bipolar disorder 53, 61–62
    Causes 62
    Lifetime risk 62
Bizarre delusions 111, 113
Bizarre mannerisms 112
Blackouts 125
Breathing exercises 28, 55, 64, 73, 74, 80, 81, 89, 90, 97, 106, 108, 118, 129, 138, 147, 156
Brief psychotic disorder 115
    Cause 115
Bulimia nervosa 136
    Causes 136
    Diagnositic criteria 136-137
    Lifetime risk 136

C

Cannabis 123
Care Approach 6
Check for signs 6–8
Civil commitment 161
Clarify safety 25
Cocaine 124
Communication skills, improving 41
Complications 124, 125
Compulsion 85, 87
Conducive atmosphere 38
Confidentiality 164-165
Crack 124
Crisis 164

Cyclothymic disorder 63
    Causes 63

D

Decisional Capacity 162
Delirium tremens 125
Delusional disorder 115–116
    Cause 116
    Lifetime risk 115
Delusions 50, 117, 118, 120, 144
Delusions, of grandeur 111
    of mind reading 111
    of reference 111
Dementia, complications 144
    Early intervention for patients 146 for caregivers 148
    Manifestations 142
Dementia of the alzheimer's type, diagnostic criteria 144-145
Dependence 126
Depression
    Changes 49
    Complications 50–51
    Early intervention for patients 55 for caregivers 57
Ddesensitization 80
Desensitization and exposure technique 30–32
Destructive behavior 24
Distractibility 60
Diversion 35, 56, 65, 73, 80, 89, 98, 117 129, 138, 156
Do's and don'ts 11
Drug abuse 122
    Complications 123
    Early intervention for patients 128 for caregivers 130
Drug dependence 122
    Complications 123
    Early intervention 128 for caregivers 130
Dysthymic disorder 53

E

Eating disorder, complications 134
Eating disorder, early intervention for caregivers 139 for patients 137
    manifestations 134
Echolalia 112
Echopraxia 112
Educate yourself 10–12
Emergency 164
Empathic gestures 41
Empathic statements 14–15, 41
Empathize generously 14
Encourage yourself 19–20
Exercise 106
Exposure 32–33, 80, 89, 90, 99

F

First aid, need for 3–4
Flight of ideas 60
Free talk 16, 41

G

Generalized anxiety disorder 104
    Causes 104
    Diagnostic criteria 104-105
    Etiology 104
    Lifetime risk 104
Anxiety disorder, psychiatric conditions 105
Grief and bereavement 154
    Early intervention for caregivers 157
    Early intervention for patients 155
    Manifestations 153
Grief, complications 153
Gustatory hallucination 111

H

Hallucinations

113, 116, 117, 118, 120, 144
HEAL technique
    10, 18, 55, 64, 72, 79, 89, 97, 106, 116, 128 137, 146, 155
Health care proxy 146
Healthy lifestyle 46
HELP method 10, 13, 66, 74, 81, 90, 99, 107, 118, 139 148, 157
Help patients 14
HELP technique 130
Help yourself 19
Heroin 125
Hierarchy 30, 33
Homicidal attempts 51, 52
Homicidal thoughts 51, 52
Hospitalization, indications 160

I

Inappropriate thoughts 34
Informed consent 162
Informed consent, exceptions 162
Intoxication 124
Involuntary hospitalization 161

L

Learn to cope 21
Listen actively 15–16
LSD 126

M

Major depressive disorder 51 52, 154
    Cause 52
    Diagnostic criteria 52-53
    Lifetime risk 52
Major depressive disorder and psychosis 52
Mania, changes 60
    Complications 61

Early intervention for caregivers 66
Early intervention for patients 64
Manic Episode, diagnostic criteria 62-63
Marijuana 123
Mastery 33
Medical conditions, weight loss 137
Memory aids 146
Mental diversion 35
Mental illness 2
Mood disorder Due to general medical condition 55
Mood disorder due to substance 64

O

Obsessions 85, 86
Obsession or Compulsion, other mental disorders 88
Obsessions and compulsions, Complications 86
    Early intervention for 89, 90
Obsessive-compulsive disorder 86 88
    Causes 87
    Diagnostic criteria 87-88
    Lifetime risk 87
Olfactory hallucination 111
Opiates 125
Outpatient clinic, indications 160

P

Panic attack, changes 69
    Complications 71
    Criteria 71
    Early intervention for patients 72 for caregivers 74
Panic attacks due to medical condition 72
Panic disorder 70

Causes 70
   Diagnostic criteria 71-72
   Lifetime risk 70
Paranoia 113
PCP 126
Persecutory delusion 111
Personal mementos 149
Phencyclidine 126
Phobia 72
Phobia, complications 77
Phobia, early intervention for
   caregivers 81
Phobia, early intervention for
   patients 79
Phobia, manifestations 77
Physical diversion 36
Physical Exercise 45
Pleasant imagery 31
Posttraumatic stress disorder 94
   96
   Lifetime risk 95
   Diagnostic criteria 95-96
   Etiology 95
Power of attorney 146
Premenstrual dysphoric disorder 54
Prevent yourself from getting sick
   17
Privilege 165
Problem-solving strategies 37, 106
Progressive muscle relaxation
   29, 55, 64, 73, 74, 80, 81
   89, 90, 97, 106, 108, 118
   129, 138, 147, 156
Psychological dependence 127
Psychosis 61
   Early intervention for
   caregivers 118
   Early intervention for patients
   116
   Manifestations 111
Psychotic disorder, medical
   condition 116

R

Recreational activities 45, 98
Red flags 7
Relaxation phase 31
Remedy 9
Respite 43
Response prevention 89, 90
Right to refuse treatment 165
Routine, escape from 43

S

Schizoaffective Disorder 63, 115
   Cause 115
Schizophrenia 113-114
   Causes 113
   Diagnostic criteria 113-114
   Lifetime risk 113
Schizophreniform, 115
   Cause 115
   Lifetime risk 115
Sedative-hypnotic-anxiolytic drugs
   126
Self-control, practice 40
Self-help groups 128
Self-help programs 130
Sign 7
Sleep hygiene 46, 56, 64, 74, 97,
   107, 118, 129, 138, 147, 156
So-what technique 73
Social diversion 36
Social phobia 72, 78
   Diagnostic criteria 78
   Lifetime risk 78
Socialization 98, 106
Specific phobia 72, 79
   Cause 79
   Lifetime risk 79
Spirituality
   46, 57, 74, 90, 99, 107, 118
   139, 148
Stigma 1
Substance abuse, diagnostic criteria

Index

128
Substance dependence, diagnostic criteria 127
Substance-induced psychotic disorder 116
Suicidal attempts 51
Suicidal behavior 123
Suicidal ideas and attempts 61
Suicidal thoughts 51
Suicidality 52
Support groups, caregivers 132
Support networks 46
Symptom 7
Systematic desensitization 30, 74, 81, 108

T

Thought blocking 112
Thought broadcasting 111
Thought disorganization 112
Thought insertion 111
Thought restructuring 34, 55, 73, 80, 89, 97, 106, 118, 138, 147, 156
Thought withdrawal 111
Time management 44
Time out 42–44
Tolerance 122, 125, 126, 127
Trauma, changes after 93
    Complications 94
Treatment failure 163

V

Vascular dementia 145
Virtual exposure 30, 33
Visual hallucination 111
Visual imagery 97
Visualization 29, 73, 74, 80, 81, 89, 106, 108

W

Will 146

Withdrawal signs and symptoms 122, 125
Wolpe, Joseph 30

Successful Preparation for the Psychiatry Oral Exam
How to Effectively Organize Your Interview, Oral Presentation, and Video Exam

Description: 184 pages, 6X9 Paperback ISBN: 0-9687816-3-2

Author: Michael G. Rayel, MD

Successful Preparation for the Psychiatry Oral Exam is written to help the psychiatry oral exam candidates effectively organize the introduction, interview, oral presentation, and video exam phases of the ABPN Part II examination. It provides detailed how-to techniques to enhance candidates' performance and improve the chance of passing this rigorous test of their competence.

Successful Preparation offers several unique features. This new book:

- Focuses on the basic and practical techniques to successfully organize the collection and presentation of data.

- Establishes the essential goals to be achieved during the exam.

- Highlights solid methodologies to start a winning introduction, obtain adequate history, and apply effective history-taking techniques.

- Offers a common sense approach toward a powerful case formulation, differential diagnosis, and treatment plan.

- Introduces several effective organizing strategies, such as the use of templates, and cassette and video recording, not commonly taught or espoused by review courses, clinical supervisors, and mock reviewers.

- Offers a practical guide to negotiating the video examination hurdle through *stop, look, and listen,* and *note-taking* strategies.

- Recognizes the common causes of disorganization and suggests ways to effectively deal with them.

- Discusses helpful methodologies in dealing with the intricacies associated with the question-and-answer portion of the exam.

- And much more!

WHAT OTHER PSYCHIATRISTS HAVE TO SAY.

"This is a practical, useful, and indispensable guide to passing part 2 of the boards, particularly for those who have not passed previously, since Dr. Rayel's common sense approach is designed to augment what many examinees do not come by intuitively or naturally."

Bernard Katz, MD
Department of Psychiatry, Harvard Medical School and Boston University School of Medicine
Chairman, Membership Committee
American Psychiatric Association

"Like an excellent supervisor, Dr. Rayel's text provides the board eligible psychiatrist with the tools necessary for passing the boards. His focused and practical approach to the task gives the reader rock solid methodology for success."

Justin O. Schecter, MD
Assistant Clinical Professor of Psychiatry
Yale University School of Medicine

For individual orders, call Soar Dime Ltd.1-866-418-7277 or fax inquiries to 709-466-2214. Now available in bookstores!

Passing Strategies: *A Helpful Guide for the Psychiatry Oral Exam*

Description: 96 pages, 6 x 9 Paperback ISBN 0-9687816-0-8
CD ISBN 0-9687816-2-4 **Cassette** ISBN 0-9687816-1-6

Author: Michael G. Rayel, MD

Passing Strategies is an indispensable companion to assist candidates in achieving success in both exam preparation and performance. Through his frank dialogue interspersed with humorous anecdotes, the author relies upon personal vignettes and the experiences of others to provide practical methods for success. Through extensive examples, the book simplifies the complexities surrounding the whole examination process.

"Michael Rayel, MD has written a textbook, guidebook, and a workbook, all in one, designed to overcome those oral board anxieties by application of the old principle, 'knowledge is power.'....This is an extremely user-friendly guidebook, which candidates will read and reread as the magic date draws closer. The no-nonsense suggestions are clear and basic and the underlying rationales, eminently sound. Beyond those points, the moral support provided by the text is extremely solid."

Thomas G. Gutheil, MD
Professor of Psychiatry
Harvard Medical School

For individual orders, call Soar Dime Ltd.1-866-418-7277 or fax inquiries to 709-466-2214. Now available in bookstores!